D0589693

4 5 0007642 0

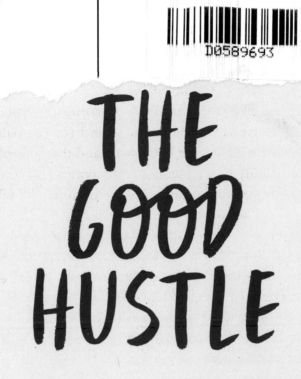

THE GOOD HUSTLE

My deepest gratitude to John McGee, without whom life would be less sweet. To the Lady Squire for bringing me into the journey. To Murwillumbah, Ubud and Portland and Brooklyn. And to my girlfriends, bhakti yogis, teachers, gurus and virtuous friends, for appearing at exactly the right time to deliver your wisdoms.

THE GOOD HUSTLE

Creating a happy, healthy
business with heart

Dr Polly McGee

MURDOCH BOOKS

SYDNEY · LONDON

Published in 2018 by Murdoch Books,
an imprint of Allen & Unwin

Text copyright © Polly McGee 2018
Photography on page 216 © Douglas Frost 2018

All rights reserved. No part of this book may be reproduced or transmitted in
any form or by any means, electronic or mechanical, including photocopying,
recording or by any information storage and retrieval system, without prior
permission in writing from the publisher. The Australian *Copyright Act 1968*
(the Act) allows a maximum of one chapter or 10 per cent of this book,
whichever is the greater, to be photocopied by any educational institution
for its educational purposes provided that the educational institution (or body
that administers it) has given a remuneration notice to the Copyright Agency
(Australia) under the Act.

Murdoch Books Australia
83 Alexander Street, Crows Nest NSW 2065
Phone: +61 (0)2 8425 0100
murdochbooks.com.au
info@murdochbooks.com.au

Murdoch Books UK
Ormond House, 26–27 Boswell Street, London WC1N 3JZ
Phone: +44 (0) 20 8785 5995
murdochbooks.co.uk
info@murdochbooks.co.uk

A catalogue record for this book is available from
the National Library of Australia

ISBN 978 1 76052 323 7 Australia
ISBN 978 1 76063 430 8 UK

Cover design by Madeleine Kane
Internal design by Vivien Valk

Printed and bound by MBM Print SCS Ltd., Glasgow

10 9 8 7 6 5 4 3 2 1

REMEMBER, YOU DON'T HAVE TO CHANGE THE WORLD, YOU JUST HAVE TO MAKE IT BETTER FOR SOMEONE ELSE FOR A MOMENT, THEN REPEAT THAT ACTION ENDLESSLY.

Contents

PART THREE: THE GOOD HUSTLE PLAYBOOK

PART FOUR: THE YOGA OF BUSINESS

Prologue: The Sacred in the Mundane

Ideas are funny things. Some of them whiz in and out, visitors that remind you of the endless store of creativity within. Others are more persistent, they are bigger and more urgent in their calls to action. Writing *The Good Hustle* was definitely one of the latter. The idea for this book came to me while I was undertaking yoga teacher training at an ashram in tropical northern New South Wales. How I came to be at that ashram was a story in itself.

By the end of 2014 I had spent a couple of years working for big organisations, in roles that should have been the crowning moments of my career. Yet I certainly didn't feel that way, and was on the point of chucking it all in and hoping I could make it working for myself. But I had niggling doubts, and was worried that I wasn't going to get enough work if I went out on my own. It came time to commit to a new contract at the place I was working. I went around in circles in my head, then decided to stay on.

A few weeks in to the new contract I knew I should have backed myself and left. But I could see the opportunity to put some behavioural change into action and make the best of my decision to stay. What if I actually tried to live each day like all of the spiritual teachings and readings recommended: in the present, surrendering the work to the divine, and seeing it as service. Aside from quitting or whingeing, I had no other option.

Each day, before I took the fifty-minute drive from my house to work, I would set an intention to simply be in the moment, to connect with everyone I met, and see how I could best serve them. Throughout this time, I was forced to admit to myself that my attachment to financial rewards and reputational standing, which I believed reflected my sense of 'value', were causing me great suffering. I had pursued careers throughout my working life that legitimised me, that showed my status, that made me authoritative, useful and 'important' in the public eye. Yet none of these careers had given me lasting happiness. The more I got, the less I had.

This suffering was self-made. I had to give up the desire for status, along with having any kind of control. It didn't change anything, except me. I began to loosen my grip, and I made it my mission to find opportunities to be of service. As a result, my world appeared more expansive, and I set about getting another project, my novel *Dogs of India*, published. I was practising discipline to make more time available to complete my paid work tasks as well as my side hustle. I had consciously begun narrowing what I put into my head: what I was reading, what I was listening to and watching. If it didn't serve my spiritual development, then I didn't fill up my mind with it.

When I look across my life with the uncensored voice of hindsight, I see that my decision-making process at that time had been run by my rampant sensory attachments with the pleasure and comfort button dialled up to ten. I believed that these sensations were what happiness was, but I couldn't get them to hang around. My rope bridge was unravelling, and I was clinging tighter and tighter to the desire for permanence. My year of living mindfully—doing something that was not my usual striving stab at pleasure followed by a swift exit before embarking on the next bite at happiness—slowed me down. It gave me time to think, to focus on what this life I had been rampaging through was all about. It gave me a taste for giving more, and doing less for my own self aggrandisement. It tuned me in to my inner wisdom. The more I listened, the more I could distinguish the sound of this spokesperson for my true self from the louder, bullying voices of its ugly sisters, self-criticism and self-doubt. I grew comfortable with my commitment to being in the moment and appreciating what I had now, not what I thought I could get around the next corner of my life.

One spring day I was driving back from a blissful yoga retreat. The weekend of meditation, kirtan, silence and yoga with one of my best friends had left me feeling a sense of deep equanimity. My spiritual practice was continuing to grow, and my gratitude and contentment along with it. Out of the blue I heard my inner voice telling me

I was done with the work I was doing, I had learned the lesson of sticking with something, and should take the next opportunity that was offered to me. The message was direct and unexpected. My last day at work was marked with a big red smiley face on my calendar and I was quite determined to complete the job. I had booked a trip to India to volunteer at a school for girls as a reward for my perseverance. But here I was, being instructed to start mentally packing my stuff in readiness for the next stage of my life. I recalibrated myself to a watching brief, curious to see what was going to happen next.

Change came, out of the blue: an offer of a short but lucrative consultancy job meant I would have enough savings to be freed from having to earn money, and could invest some time in developing my own projects. At the same time, a fortuitous conversation had lead to a publishing deal for *Dogs of India*. Surrendering, listening to my inner voice, working from a place of divinity, asking for help was delivering. I felt happy, fulfilled and motivated. In late December, as I was preparing for my imminent departure to India, a small ad popped up in my Facebook feed for a two-month immersion yoga teacher training at a spiritual community set in an ashram near Byron Bay.

I instantly knew without question that I had to go, that this was the experience that was calling me to prepare myself for the next adventure of my life and I should cancel my other plans. Even with my appetite for agile life decisions, this one was left field. I decided to listen to my inner guide again and back my intuition. I cancelled my trip to India and headed north to the ashram.

In so many things I do, I compare my approach to that of a method actor, diving in and living in character, Stanislavski style. Now, it appeared, I was going to become a yogi. But not your live-in-a-cave-style yogi. I was going to be an urban yogi, living a life with meaning and joy, though integrating the traditional restraints and observances of yogi life. When I talk about being yogi throughout this book, it is a metaphor for a life where you are pointing yourself towards something bigger than you are. Something with meaning that motivates grit and resilience in pursuing your goals to get to your higher self. But being yogi doesn't happen overnight. I had to get ready. On 1 January I gave up meat, fish, eggs and booze in preparation for ashram life. By diving in with only four weeks to get my practice on, I didn't have time to think about the social impacts of this radical change of lifestyle, whether people would judge me or think I wasn't fun anymore. I had such an attachment to being a foodie and my cork-popping, cocktail-shaking life, and if I'd overthought it, I definitely would have struggled, suffered and faltered. Instead, I just became yogi, and so all my choices followed this new path of living. It was easy to say no, because I knew how hard it would be if I went to the ashram unprepared mentally for the physical demands. By being what I wanted to become, I became it. In Buddhism, you meditate on the Buddha as though you possess all of the qualities of a fully enlightened being and behave with complete compassion. You aren't the Buddha—yet. But in doing this practice you are acknowledging that within all of us there is Buddha nature: the capacity for enlightenment in this lifetime.

It is much easier to do nothing if you feel there is no way you can reach the finish line. By acknowledging what's possible, finding the sacred in the mundane—the daily acts that stitch our days, weeks and lives together—I set my mind to living the right way, accepting that there would be plenty of wrong paths taken along the journey. This undoubtedly accelerated and deepened my spiritual experience. It also became my earliest foray into growth mindset.

The decision to take two months out to live yogi after a life of striving was life changing. The experience of being completely immersed in spirituality, spending hours each day practising yoga, reading ancient spiritual texts, meditating, chanting mantra, living as a yogi in service to all sentient beings—it was home. I'd always thought it sounded really corny when people say that, but what it means is that we feel what it is like to be our true selves. I felt like my inner voice was sitting on a rock by the river's edge, gently asking what took me so long.

I'd found my dharma—what it meant to give value and feel I was the essence of me. I don't mean being a yoga teacher, or any specific task, but immersing myself in spirituality, in a practical everyday sense. I had been drawn to Eastern spirituality and philosophy since I was a child. But I'd had no outlet to explore that in the non-religious household I grew up in, and no role models to guide me. This is an important point on how we find our paths. It can be hard to know how to apply something you read in a book to your own life. Author, academic and yogi Stephen Cope describes finding your tribe as encountering 'a full expression of kindred dharma'. That's a nice way to think of those role models. Watching someone else blossom is the trigger for our own inner seeds to germinate. Hence the need to find those teachers, and Sangha, to surround yourself with a spiritual cheer squad to help you grow. Living in dharma, living with meaning and applying the eight limbs of yoga to my own life had a profound impact on my happiness. I stopped looking outwards to everything and everyone for validation and approval, stopped trying to be the best and the smartest, and went within to try to build some discipline in my own mind.

The eight weeks at the ashram, and the month before that, when I started being yogi, and the year before that, when I had consciously practised discipline and faith in the surrender, were the beginning of a year of confidently following my heart and mind, rather than being wagged by the tail of reaction and attachment.

Perhaps it was my experience working with entrepreneurs and start-ups that made the connection between the eight-limbed path of yoga and the journey of the entrepreneur appear so logical. There seemed an absolute synergy between the two missions and when the idea of combining the two as a method of building heart-centred businesses came to me, I couldn't unsee it.

The coupling kept popping up, and the deeper I dug during my immersion in the ashram and the weeks that followed, the more I read, the more I sat and thought, the more it resonated that when the desire to do something bigger was overlayed with the motivation driving entrepreneurial and business activities, a powerful union emerged. Further study of the teachings of the Buddhadharma pointed to a new model of spiritually embodied business behaviour and leadership. It became clear to me that once the mind was understood through the discipline of meditation and self-study advocated in the ancient yogic texts, the approach to business could be liberated from some of the attachment and suffering entrepreneurs looking to establish heart-centred business ventures often felt.

Like many of my clients, I want to be part of enterprises that have a bigger motivation than money and success. Sure, those things are great by-products, but for me, I want to really love my projects because I see and feel the impacts the work is having on others. I want to be of service to all sentient beings, not just humans, but animals, plants, the ocean and earth, from massive to tiny—all matter matters. Sometimes that alone is the reason to begin something, rather than a profit motive. In a world where even the best business ideas with a sure-fire market trajectory can (should and do) fail, the idea of starting up an enterprise or taking a role based on being of service, values and love isn't that crazy. You may have come to this book with an idea for a business, service or product, but not know how to go about bringing it to fruition. Or you may have a longing for change in your life, and picked this up looking for some pointers on how to identify what it is you want to do, ready to get going when the lightning strikes. Either way, you are preparing the ground of your mind as a fertile environment to seed an idea and bring it to fruition.

If you have a yearning in life, a restlessness in your consciousness that you feel is unmet, this book is for you. It's not a book that seeks to balance your work or life, it's a book about the totality of us, and what we are and do and why. It's not a book that will spit out a business plan at the end, or give you endless templates and tick-box quizzes to execute. There is already a mountain of excellent resources available in the virtual and real world to help you with those tasks. Nor is this a book of spiritual materialism and positive-thinking-driven personal development, although I am going to spend as much, if not more, time focusing on you as I am on the business. This is a book that I hope will give you the most important tool of all—an understanding of the role your mind plays in the way you experience the world and who you are driven to serve. It will help you discover what that might look and feel like, and how you can scale your new focus into a marketable idea to create a good hustle business, or be present in and for your organisation and co-workers. *The Good Hustle* is a book to help bridge the gap for many of us who identify with a spiritual path, and who don't see that path as separate to our work, but as the centre of everything we do.

If I was to create a persona of the person likely to pick up this book, it would look something like this: you've spent some time, probably a lot of time and no doubt with significant investment, on various journeys of self-discovery. Perhaps this has been to improve a singular element of your life: love, money, career or health for example. Or perhaps it was because you had a niggling feeling that you weren't complete.

You have a fundamental desire to change the way you feel about yourself. You may also want to change that thing you do to earn an income stream so it aligns with the totality of you and your values. You are probably juggling myriad responsibilities and activities, some intellectual, some physical, some emotional (some hormonal). And you have an interior space that is locked down, blocked up, a chair against the door of your self; where the parts of you that are your greatest critic ferment happily, bubbling to the surface when you least need to hear them.

Which is, of course, constantly.

This self-critical dialogue has been part of what might be holding you back from pushing ahead with your business idea, even though you have a killer idea and a gut feeling that you just need to do it and the time is right. You need some tools, you need some straight-up advice, you need some support for your internal emotional compass, and you don't want to be sold to, patronised, mansplained, or assaulted by the subtle aggression of self-development gurus. If this is you, then we are in the right place, at the right time, and this is the right book.

I want to show you the tap that turns on the flow of all of the good things into your being: the sparkle, the creativity, the frisson of authenticity, the step full of spring for your idea. I want to take your ideas out of the 'too hard' basket and drop them into the one labelled 'Let's *do* this'. I want you to find the effortlessness of self-love and fulfilment, of being not doing. I want you to give benefit to others as your default setting, and sign off on a permanent permission note to being enough. Working on and in business where the hustle is inherently good is a pathway to achieving some of that. It's business, it's a way of being, but it's also who you are, and so throughout the text I'm going to weave in some personal insights to illustrate the experience.

The method acting of being yogi has become my lifestyle. Whenever I begin to worry about things I can't control, or find myself making endless future plans, I stop, and focus on what I'm doing at that moment, reminding myself to leave everything else alone. I try to do my dharma day after day, and the feeling of general equanimity prevails. It doesn't stop the suffering when things happen to trip you up, but it puts the suffering in context for the long game of this life. You don't hold on to the trip and make it a big drama. You get up, laugh and point to the mud all over you and keep going. It is the kind of suffering you are happy to fight for and endure, knowing it is impermanent.

Saying no comes much easier to me now. I don't worry about my reputation, or whether people like me, or if my decisions are going to make other people happy. Each choice is made through the lens of service and I just do what I do with as much compassion and love as I can muster, and work towards mustering more. The reduction in highs and lows means that there is so much more productive time in the day. I'm not saying the occasional nap doesn't slip in, but it's a conscious rest, rather than an escape from the world. There's no longer a desire to numb out pain with food, booze and other experiential pleasures, so I save plenty of money, which means I can devote more time to creativity for the sake of good hustle and not simply to make money at all costs. I have all the riches I need, with no requirement to look outside.

The Good Hustle is a book all about you and me, and us and them as one. It is also a book about being and becoming the best you can be, and measuring this with simple metrics, like your capacity to love, serve and connect. So, welcome to *The Good Hustle*, a revelation and revolution combining the ancient wisdoms of yogis and Buddhas with the contemporary genius of living and working in a lean, agile, heart-centred way.

Introduction

Becoming 'awake'
involves seeing our confusion
more clearly.

CHÖGYAM TRUNGPA, BUDDHIST MONK,
MEDITATION MASTER AND AUTHOR

Australian palliative care nurse Bronnie Ware, in her book *The Top Five Regrets of the Dying*, says that the number one regret her dying patients express is the wish to have had more courage to live a life true to themselves, not the life others expected of them. The words sound easy, but the application of them, once we start to unpack the ideas, is incredibly difficult. If we are true to our authentic desire, what is it that we want? Once the question is posed, we need to begin the hunt within for the answers. And we need to be really brave in pursuing our own truths. The deeper we look inside, and begin to know who we really are and honour that knowledge, the more we'll aspire to do what is most beneficial, and the greater courage we'll have to make the right choices—for us and others.

So here are the questions we are going to pose as we start this adventure together: what if we are enough just as we are? What if there is no need to strive, to achieve, to crush the opposition, to get to the top, or to succeed in that traditional way of measurable gains? What if our sense of self is the sense that all we are is part of a greater whole? What if we can create heart-centred businesses or enterprises that allow us to do something we love, that are sustainable and viable and serve the market and our customers to our and their higher good? What if we could pursue endeavours that also leave us feeling well, not exhausted, stressed and anxious? And the big existential what if: what if there isn't a destination to happiness that comes from striving and doing, what if everything is simply a continuum of curiosity and becoming? These questions and hypotheses will be tested throughout this book by combining the practice of creating lean start-ups with the ancient wisdoms found in the teachings of yoga and meditation. Not a combination usually found in MBA or small business courses, but one far more common than you would think in the practice of entrepreneurs who understand that all transactions happen in the mind before they happen in the marketplace. The book is structured in four sections. The first, Heart Centred, tackles the tension of combining spirituality with business, and the shadow issue of our own deep-seated lack, and the fear that holds us hostage. Once we have begun the conversation with ourselves, it's time to look for our innate good hustle motivation in Part Two, Desperately Seeking Dharma: an investigation of the idea of dharma and how we can best deliver service to others throughout our lives. Part Three is where we 'be it till we are it' with The Good Hustle Playbook: a bundle of mindful business practices you can use to conceive and implement your good hustle. And finally, in Part Four, we travel along the path to enlightenment with The Yoga of Business: an application of lean start-up principals aligned to the Yoga Sutras and Buddhism's eight worldly dharmas as a way of preparing to launch your sustainable, successful good hustle into the world.

I believe in applying the practice of yoga holistically. With a simple set of disciplined practices, yoga can disarm the nuclear arsenal of our self-critical minds and reactive behaviours, turning them (and us) into powerful forces for good. While we have adopted yoga asana practice in the West, and are now beginning to see the significant impact a physical practice can have, there is a need to apply the full expression of yoga to the places where we concentrate so much of the effort and energy of our lives, like our careers. We need to be able to create those fleeting moments of calm that we experience on the mat or the cushion, and infuse them into our twenty-four hour days. We need to visit or revisit the fundaments of yoga as a system of knowledge for navigating being human and apply it systematically and holistically, so we live yogi, and that includes the yoga of business. Meditation similarly fits within the practice of yoga, in fact it is inextricable from both the eight-limbed yogi's path and every step of Buddha's eightfold path.

Yoga and Buddhism in the West are positioned not as 'religions' but as systems of philosophical interrogation and practice. Yoga is, however, still a system deriving from the Hindu religion and is closely connected with all aspects of Hindu dharma and much of Indian culture. Buddhism also shares many similarities with religion, even though the Dalai Lama often refers to it as a science or philosophy.

Today, yoga is most known for its asanas, or postures, which are the most visible and outward form of the system. Buddhism is known as a tradition of meditation, as in the more popular forms of Buddhist meditation like Zen and Vipassana. This is a quirk of the West that says more about us and how we have interpreted these disciplines than it does about the true nature of yoga, which is traditionally defined as meditation, or calming the disturbances of the mind, not as asana, which is taught merely as an aid to meditation. I'm giving you this micro version of the roots of yoga and Buddhism to set up where most of us will be in our interpretations and understandings of the vast body of yogic and Buddhist teachings. You don't need to be a purist, or a hybridist, or an any-ist to get the gist of how they are going to be incorporated into your path of enlightenment in the good hustle. If you're not a cat who's sat on a mat—yoga or meditation—you are still perfectly prepared for what comes next. If you have a deep belief in a Christian, Jewish, Hindu or Muslim God(s) or are a raging atheist, then you are likewise not going to be excluded or offended by *The Good Hustle* and its view on incorporating your version of spirituality into your business idea and merging both into a life that is healthy, happy and full of heart.

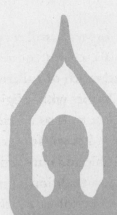

PART ONE

HEART CENTRED

This is the age of doing work that matters...
if you feel like what you do doesn't
make an impact, no amount of money
will keep you there.

GALA DARLING, AUTHOR, SPEAKER, INTERNATIONAL PLAYGIRL

THE BUSINESSES I'M TALKING ABOUT ARE
DESIGNED AROUND LOVE AND DEVOTION
TO CUSTOMERS, AROUND BEING IN SERVICE.
YOU AREN'T TRYING TO MANIFEST A
DIAMOND NECKLACE TO BRING HAPPINESS,
YOU ARE POLISHING THE DIAMOND OF YOUR
ESSENTIAL SELF TO FIND THE CONTENTMENT
THAT COMES FROM LIVING HOLISTICALLY.

The God of Small (Business) Things

Business and spirituality aren't separate. I want to address this issue at the start, as it is something that I struggled to articulate clearly to myself for a long period of time. The same awkwardness that can arise when trying to find the words to express your version of God or the divine is amplified when mixed in with the often undivine world of work and business. There is a widely spread belief that spiritual businesses are the evolution of what used to be called 'New Age' businesses, which in itself now seems a kooky and antiquated term. New Age was code for some kind of tie-dyed hippy enterprise that was floating around in the ether dripping with crystals and fairy dust and certainly not rooted in any serious or robust business practice. The New Age business was kryptonite to the Gordon Gekko mode of business in the eighties, where money was the underpinning of an era built on ego, assets and ruthless acquisitions. The reaction to the soulless and exploitative nature of that time in Western culture was the emergence of the spiritual and motivational movement, where the icons of merging success with a higher purpose were emerging empowerment celebrities Tony Robbins and Oprah Winfrey.

With mainstream media-savvy champions, spirituality got a makeover, one where success and soulfulness could coexist and still maintain the razzle-dazzle of a sales convention where everyone was a winner. Positive thinking and speaking prevailed. This is a very loose and anecdotal timeline of the cultural progression of how a certain view of spirituality was embedded in our understanding. Without doubt, the most significant contribution to having your cake and manifesting it too was the publication of *The Secret* by Rhonda Byrne. A book, and then movie, that not only told us we could be spiritual, but also gave us permission to use the mystical power of the Universe to provide us with endless material wealth.

This idea played beautifully into the fear of not being or having enough, in a world addicted to instant gratification and consumption. *The Secret* taught us that we could manifest anything if we were clear on our intention, and handed over control to the Universe, which was inferred to be a massive energetic Walmart that would spontaneously deliver our hearts' desires. Of course, this was simply more of what renegade monk and author Chögyam Trungpa would disparagingly call 'material spiritualism'. It was Gordon Gekko manifested through the longing for possessions to fill the well of emptiness so many people felt. *The Secret* spawned an enormous sector of spiritual marketers who took the manifesting business to new heights of aspiration with billions of dollars in book sales and workshop revenues.

This movement also built a concept of happiness based around more stuff—more of the things that are, in my belief, the cause of so much of our present-day suffering. It portrayed personal happiness as the result of personal acquisition, not as the result of giving and working towards the happiness of others. The work needed was all pointed outwards, and because of that, there was an all-care-no-responsibility clause: if the happiness that all those other manifestors had found didn't miraculously appear in your driveway, round your neck or on your finger, it was because *you* were doing it wrong. Which of course for so many people was an inbuilt short cut to failure, anxiety and proof of not being enough. And the cycle of material life continued. What better snake oil to sell to a culture gorging on possessions and status than a brand of spirituality that netted more possessions and status. Genius, right? A couple of decades later, there is an increasing awareness that our mass consumption is having a serious impact on people and the environment, and there is more suffering around than ever. We are looking for connection, for compassion and for meaning that is beyond the individual, and a desire to connect that with our own spirituality.

The central message of *The Good Hustle* is that *all* business and work can be conducted in a way that connects the action with what we can describe as something bigger than you. It doesn't have to be a spiritual business, you don't have to be a yogi or a vegan raw foodist, or live in a blue zone to be of benefit. (Although you may well be rocking the pants out of that lifestyle. If so, all power to you.) I'm not insisting on you accessorising or purchasing anything to get started (except this book of course, but you know libraries are free!). The purpose of integrating spiritual teachings and lean start-up principals is giving you the capacity to create a business, enterprise, organisation, venture, co-op or, for that matter, job that makes you feel motivated, joyful and connected. For this to be sustainable, if you aren't heading straight to a cave and accepting offerings into a bowl, you need to be able to create enough revenue for the business to survive and thrive, and you (and your staff) along with it. To do so, you need to have built your good hustle on the foundation of a realistic and measurable market that needs what you are offering at a price that covers costs and that you meet (and hopefully exceed) the expectation of your customers. The rules are the rules are the rules when it comes to the equation that enables sustainable growth, whether spirituality is present in your business plan or not. *Opportunity + meeting sufficient market demand + sale = revenue.*

But loudly, proudly and unashamedly, the differentiator is that the businesses I'm talking about are designed around love and devotion to customers, around being in service. You aren't trying to manifest a diamond necklace to bring happiness, you are polishing the diamond of your essential self to find the contentment that comes from living holistically. This life of joy and meaning all happens in the world as we know it, not in a mythical place where the stresses and strains of your life disappear, the children are quiet and angelic, the traffic flows and your groceries miraculously appear in the pantry. It's the same old life, same old world, same old issues, but with a radically revisioned approach to how you react to them. It's not just business that will become spiritual, it's everything that you do, all juiced up to be of service to others.

No need to rush out and burn your vision board, kids. The repetitive themes and longings of your life will provide rich clues to where you are heading if you currently feel rudderless. Spoiler alert—your vision board will not end up a catalogue of future purchases and status symbols. The success of your good hustle will not be measured by the number of zeroes in your bank balance. It will be felt in your heart, and in your connection with the infinite amount of sentient beings, human and other, that you are unconditionally loving through your work. Ain't no vision board big enough to accurately represent that.

Growing Pains

What do you want to be when you grow up? What do you want to do? Familiar questions—most, if not all, of us have been confronted with a request to select our futures on demand. Perhaps in high school, when you were trying to decide which elective class would define your entire future. Or perhaps even earlier, when parents and relatives were forensically searching for clues as to which of your childhood whims might transform into a career.

When I was really young, I wanted to be a writer. My first book, lovingly hand bound by my mother, was about a dog that had a tongue made of bacon. I was obviously ahead of the curve as a four-year-old, intuitively understanding the bacon zeitgeist even then. At seven I wanted to be a 'lady of the night', as it was euphemistically referred to in my family. It seemed a very appealing career choice at that age, to be allowed to get all dressed up with epic hair and makeup and no one telling you to go to bed at 7 p.m. And you could have tattoos. I would secretly pack a bag at night, and lie in bed planning my escape to Kings Cross (where I knew the night ladies hung out) with its bright lights and what seemed to be limitless potential for adventure.

From my earliest memories I coveted tattoos, and marvelled at those dudes and (occasionally) dames who were allowed to have them, and their effortless cool. In my family they were strictly denounced as the denominator of 'commonness' and vice. I had no idea of what a prostitute did or what sex even was. The envious and innocent pre-Internet child that was me interpreted those women as free spirits, out late at night without their parents, expressing themselves on their own terms. Feminists, if you will. Everything I wasn't at age seven.

I admit these were a pretty kooky set of goals and observations of the world around me, and the travails of sex work were completely beyond my young mind. Without any kind of reality filter, however, I was obviously drawn to an embodied world of service (and aesthetics.) As I hit my teens, the other career I really wanted to pursue was hairdressing (again, service, aesthetics, cool hair *and* tattoo opportunities, but no sex required). Like my other work aspirations, Mum shut this down vigorously on the 'too common' ground. Don't get me wrong. This wasn't a mean-spirited, killjoy motif. Like most parents, what Mum wanted for me was a life and education better than her own.

I was raised to believe I could have and do anything I put my mind to, and the scaffolding of this was education as emancipation. Obediently taking on the values and beliefs of my parents, this is where I undoubtedly began my decades-long tussle with identifying and living my dharma versus doing what I believed others thought was right for me in order to please them.

What we do is a significant part of how we describe ourselves, and herein lies one of the fundamental problems of our time. If we aren't our work and our incomes, our status and our ambitions, our ownership and our achievements, who and what are we—and what is our purpose? In recent years this question has shifted into another loaded way of asking what you want to be when you grow up: what is your Passion, with a capital P? Or sometimes, your equally capitalised Purpose?

Passion and Purpose are, quite frankly, another sneaky way of asking about the nature of who we are, defined externally through what we do (and what status that confers). Passion is personal. It is something we really should know, the inference being otherwise we are lacking a lust for life, or something more fundamental. Another lucrative industry has emerged around helping people to find their Passion and Purpose through various self-styled self-help gurus. And in the words of Alanis Morissette, 'Isn't it ironic?' Who better to be able to know what it is we love and are passionate about than us, and not some external party? (Double Alanis points for irony if you have noted that this is also a book that you had to purchase about helping you find your Passion and Purpose.)

But as we think we are not enough, we look to (and pay) others to do the big reveal on ourselves. The real irony is that we won't speak, hear or act on our truths while we are caught in an endless cycle of internal criticism, comparison and invalidation of our ideas. Our passions are muted by deep longings for love, acceptance and understanding from outside. I know now my childhood careers were not the path to happiness and self-realisation I thought they were, but there were elements in that mini-me wisdom of what motivates me to this day. There was no one in my family, neighbourhood or community that modelled a life I aspired to. That spiritual kin I mentioned in the beginning of the book were missing in guiding and validating my choices. I had no idea what I wanted to be, although I was very clear on the type of career and higher education others thought would be suitable for me. If only I had known then that I shouldn't have been searching for a title on a business card. I should have been looking for a feeling, a sense of wellbeing, a jigsaw piece slipping snugly into its hole as a clue to my true nature of self.

Those of us who can only give a vague wish list of our Passions and Purpose, or worse, who have no firm answer or who want to do things with no visible commercial outcomes, like be an artist or musician, often find ourselves viewed as second-class doers. Subordinate to a class of people who were born with a vocational spoon in their mouths, destined for something definable somewhere—with a clear economic benefit. I violently envied those people who effortlessly knew what they wanted, no shadows of doubt. Just a clear runway to self-actualisation.

The worst thing about big P questions, when unable to be swiftly and surely answered, is that they cause real anxiety. I remember vividly the rising panic I felt through most of my twenties and early thirties as I searched for my purpose like I was ransacking a sale bin. I tried on career after career, experiencing a brief euphoria as I convinced myself that I had finally found my Purpose and Passion, then I'd quickly crash with the bleak realisation that whatever job I was doing was just as flawed and unsatisfying as everything else I'd done. And I'd done a lot. Just in case you thought I was some kind of quitter, here is a selection of the jobs I have wholeheartedly thrown myself into since launching my adult life of finding my dharma: chef, hairdresser, sandwich hand, commercial shopfitter, window-dresser, fashion retailer, call centre agent, cafe owner, adult film reviewer, political lobbyist, digital strategist, farmhand, artist-in-residence, radio presenter, public servant, speechwriter, innovation grants manager, IP manager, not-for-profit co-founder, copywriter, web builder, academic, author, yoga teacher, social media trainer, strategic marketing lead.

It was indeed a watershed moment as I scraped the bottom of that sales bin and finally surrendered to perhaps never knowing what my Purpose was, and that this ignorance was okay. Surrender instantly made me feel better and lighter. I didn't need to know my Passion and Purpose. I just had to enjoy what I was doing right now. Just focus on the task at hand. A frayed knot of beliefs and self-criticism unravelled with the simple epiphany that I was spending all my time yearning for a future that didn't exist. Worrying over it, building a complex second life around, well, nothing, while flagrantly squandering the life I was living in the pursuit of a hypothetical future life. Dumb, right? Plus—if I didn't have to do this mythical 'something' that was my Passion and Purpose, well, I could actually do anything. The world opened up as I awakened to my potential.

Getting a lot of tattoos also helped.

That sounds a little glib, but in truth the one constant since my childhood has been this inexplicable love of tattoos. And not just a small, discreet rose on a buttock never to be seen by the world. I wanted lots and lots of tattoos, everywhere. While everything else I was striving for seemed elusive and meaningless, as I kept striving, I rebelled against my own internal critic who cautioned me that making permanent inky choices would spell disaster when I finally happened upon my one true career that demanded a clean and proper body. That scared voice, it's fair to say, lost the battle.

And inadvertently I won the war.

By marking myself permanently, in an act of celebration, I reminded myself every day who I essentially was and had been for as long as I could remember. Let me reiterate that this was a completely unconscious act—you couldn't have found a less self-aware, mostly self-loathing human than I was in my twenties. But as my arms and other bits became more colourful and covered, I inhabited the skin I was in, and because of this, I pushed myself into career places that I had always been told tattooed women would never be allowed. This all seems a little hard to fathom now when you see an endless stream of proud tattooed women in all walks of life.

When I first started out, especially working in rural and regional Australia, I saw myself as a self-appointed spokesmodel for the tattooed woman. I believed I could be an ambassador for the skills, professionalism and compassion of my people—reversing the images and stereotypes I had grown up with of tattooed people as criminal ne'er-do-wells. And thus, in the most confounding and roundabout way, I set myself on the path of a life of service, of being an exemplar. I should have read the good hustle playbook about getting the self-love part down pat first, before I forged out on my mission, but hindsight is a fairly useless skill for living in the moment.

Grow Your Brain

There is one more fairly significant discovery I made that I believe freed me from the cycle of striving and disappointment, and that was learning a concept known as 'growth mindset'. Growth mindset straddles applied psychology and educational theory. I was introduced to it when I was doing some research for a start-up edtech company that was building educational programs for preschool kids. I was tasked with cataloguing all of the research that had been globally undertaken on the topic, and me being me, I not only catalogued, I read a lot of it as well. And it completely blew my mind.

I mentioned earlier how surrendering to the realisation that I should stop my fruitless search for my Purpose brought on a massive sense of relief—I didn't have to know what it was, I could do anything. I didn't realise it at the time, but right there I had had my very own growth mindset moment. So what is it? The concept of a growth mindset was developed by psychologist and Stanford University professor Carol Dweck through her research programs, and book *Mindset: The New Psychology of Success*. Growth mindset research and in-class testing over many years demonstrated a major positive change to learning capacity in children (and adults) who applied a growth mindset instead of a fixed mindset to their process of learning and skills acquisition. This change was a direct result of being taught the tools to approach tasks using a mindset that encouraged elements like collaboration, experimentation, effort and failure as integral to the learning journey. People will differ in their initial talents and aptitudes, interests or temperaments, but everyone can change and grow through application and experience. Having a growth mindset isn't just learning related. It also has a profound effect on personal relationships, professional success and many other dimensions of life. The greater impacts of growth mindset on creating mentally resilient children who in turn become mentally resilient adults is why it is so important to teach growth mindset thinking as early as possible, and incorporate it into a child's approach to learning and living.

A mindset, according to Professor Dweck's definition, is a self-perception that people hold about themselves and the larger world. Holding the belief that you are intelligent or unintelligent is a simple example of a mindset. People may also have a mindset related to their personal or professional lives, a fixed binary or bias like being good or bad at a task or role.

In the fixed mindset worldview, individuals believe that basic personal traits and situations, like talent and intellect, are permanent states, and these are predetermined markers of success. You either have talent, or you don't. If, for instance, you believe you are 'dumb' at certain things, say maths or language learning, you won't attempt them, and continue to perpetuate the idea (and subsequent reality) of that belief. Conversely, with a fixed mindset worldview, if you do have a particular skill or talent, this has to be maintained at all costs, and needs to be proven to the world over and over, causing stress and anxiety from striving to maintain the status quo, rather than further exploring, developing or growing that skill set.

The antidote to the fear-based, limited approach of fixed mindset is adopting a growth mindset. With a growth mindset, people believe that *effort* creates talent, and skills are learned over time, through trial and error. The capacity to 'positively' fail, where individuals learn from their mistakes and use that learning as a plank of mental growth towards achieving the skill, is a key difference in the growth mindset approach. Strongly underpinning growth mindset is resilience or grit. As learning a new skill takes time and will inevitably involve setbacks along the way, resilience and perseverance need to be developed and sustained. Students who use a growth mindset approach have been shown to learn more and embrace challenges and failures enthusiastically as opportunities rather than setbacks.

Instead of relentlessly hammering them with the idea of finding Passion and Purpose, we should instead be indoctrinating children into learning the art of a growth mindset. I support Professor Dweck's implication that a fixed mindset is the default for most people, and add to it my belief that institutions like schools and universities strongly perpetuate the idea that talent is somewhat inherent and needs to be amplified rather than grown from scratch. In my own experience, I was told from a young age at school and at home that I had no skill in maths or science and basically shouldn't bother pursuing them. In the fixed mindset worldview, my talents were in the softer skills of English and home economics, so I abandoned all efforts at numbers, and instead made it my mission to be the best at the things I could already do. I imagine now what it would have been like if instead of being told I had no skill, I was told I had no skill . . . yet, and that as I appeared to be struggling with maths, I should look for a different approach to working out the problems. This is the genius of growth mindset; it tells you not to give up, and that you don't have to know the answer, you have to find the answer. And you will, in time, with effort. The other sneaky boomerang about having a fixed mindset is that the things you are good at, your god-given talent as it were, have to be demonstrated over and over and over for the rest of your life. The theory being that if you fail at the few things you excel at, you are *really* a failure. A perfect example of seeing this play out in life is with professional athletes. So often they have been identified as talented in their particular discipline in childhood, and told their whole life they are special because of this one attribute. It defines them, and so when their careers end, they find themselves unable to forge a satisfying or fulfilling life after sport, and in some cases, the consequences are disastrous. They simply haven't acquired the skills of a growth mindset, which would enable them to ask: what's next, how can I grow my brain now? When you apply this type of thinking to the Passion and Purpose dilemma, it gets a lot simpler. If you can learn to do anything with determination and sheer hard work, then your Passion is in maintaining that curiosity. If your Passion for work is in giving and being of service or benefit, working for others and creating your happiness through that prism, that can be applied to any action from the most mundane to the most significant. That would change the whole childhood conversation, from what do you want to be when you grow up, to who do you want to benefit?

Work. What is it Good For?

It is an unspoken and intrinsically accepted part of contemporary First World culture that nearly all of us have a point of entry into the workforce, however that job is defined. We then spend the majority of our lifetime 'doing', to generate wealth for ourselves and our families to fund the ever-escalating task of living comfortably (or for many, simply to survive).

Apple founder the late Steve Jobs famously said, 'You've got to find what you love . . . Your work is going to fill a large part of your life, and the only way to be truly satisfied is to do what you believe is great work. And the only way to do great work is to love what you do.' He has his own Alanis Morissette moment of irony: Jobs was renowned as a terrifying and intimidating tyrannical boss who sent many an idealistic employee into deep states of despair after thinking that a job at Apple with one of the world's best-known entrepreneurs was the answer to their quest for Passion and Purpose.

And therein lies the rub. Our education from an early age points us towards attaining knowledge and skills to work for and in *someone else's* business. Rarely are you groomed to think independently, entrepreneurially, to win and lose and lose and win, knowing that this is all part and parcel of the rich and gratifying impermanence of taking your ideas to market. Instead, we learn compliance, dependence, subservience, the rule of control and command. We learn how to fit in, and in many cases disappear, with a reliable income; endless acquisition of stuff and status being traded for finding ourselves. Did someone say fixed mindset environment?

How are you feeling right now reading this—is this empty striving part of your reality? Are you feeling all defensive about your choice of a salaried, mortgaged life and the pinch of golden handcuffs? Don't get me wrong: this is the reality for most of us. In Buddhism it is said that we are all born with an awakened state of mind, known as Buddha nature. Wisdom, love, kindness and compassion are our true natures of being. Frustration, jealousy, guilt, shame, anxiety, greed, competitiveness and so on are experiences we learn through the influences of our culture, our families, education and our friends. These notions are then reinforced by personal experience. It is a universally applied affliction that we have to work hard to firstly have awareness of, and then harder to reverse. My criticism here is that we are groomed for suffering and attachment from infancy. We are taught how to look for the title and career that will define us, and we literally pay for it for the rest of our lives. This is the Buddhist definition of samsara, and it is the condition of being human.

From the earliest stages of our lives, our innate hunches about what brings us time-stands-still joy, and triggers an understanding of who we are, are influenced by accepted norms. We have to grow up, we have to be stable, we have to have and do a job, and eventually we have to own a house, acquire a partner and continue on the race for status. This is our broad span of normative benchmarks, from which deviation is not celebrated and championed, until success is well and truly established. Few people are cheering in the corner of the gal or guy who quits their salaried job to pursue a crazy idea to change the world through love and humanity. In my clients' experience, one of the great motivators for starting a business or pursuing a creative idea is to transition work from being an unlovable drudge to something that catapults you out of bed into a day (and often night) of empowered, satisfying activity. The love part that Steve Jobs talks of is unquestionably one of the perfect metaphors relating to work and your own venture. In love's full sense of being unconditional it encompasses the joyfulness and the drudgery, the highs and the horrors, and mediates them all with the sense of total acceptance of any situation. And right here, in the words of Steve Jobs and in my own break-up with the search for a Purpose, is where the good hustle merges with the yoga of business.

Yoga to the People

If you have only encountered yoga as physical postures or asana in a yoga class, then it's time to meet the bigger yoga family—just a brief introduction, as we will be spending plenty of quality time with yoga and its eight limbs later in this book. Yoga's history is somewhat mysterious due to the oral transmission of many of its sacred texts and the secretive nature of its teachings. What we know is that yoga can be traced back over 5000 years, and that as a science it has evolved and continues to have relevance across cultures through innovation, practice and development. With origins in Northern India, the word yoga was first mentioned in a sacred text called the Rig Veda. The Vedas were a collection of texts containing songs, mantras and rituals to be used by Brahmans, the Vedic priests. The most renowned of the yogic scriptures is the Bhagavad Gita, composed around 500 BC. The Yoga Sutras, written by Patanjali, were the first systematic presentation of yoga, breaking it down into an eight-limbed path pointing seekers to the stages of obtaining 'samadhi' or enlightenment. Patanjali was never keen on the Sutras being viewed as a definitive, prescriptive work. Rather, he saw the eight limbs as an evolution in collaboration with other sages and yogis. Obviously, a totally growth mindset kinda guy and a lover of the minimum viable product methodology (more on that later). Systems of yoga continued to be developed in India through the exploration of physical and spiritual connections and body-focused practices, which became known as hatha yoga—this is the principal yoga we know and practise in the West. Patanjali's eight limbs of yoga, being a foundation from which to explore rather than a finite set of rules, still offer a completely relevant and logical pathway for self-discovery. The pathway isn't necessarily linear, and each element offers insights in recalibrating how we work with meaning and live with joy.

Introducing the Hustlepedia

There are a couple of words and concepts I've already used that need to be defined here, as they are variously interpreted, and have quite specific meanings in the context of creating a good hustle. Their definitions may be different from how you currently use and understand them.

OMG

Let's start with the big one first, so all mentions of creator, source, higher power, faith, divinity, God or whomever, are able to be moulded to your particular belief system.

I'm the first to acknowledge that I struggled with this for years. Not having come from a family that had any kind of faith, my overwhelming thoughts about the big G God that I saw in Christian traditions was that this concept was totally unrelatable to me.

The first rule of *The Good Hustle* is there is no one, dominant belief system. Whatever your perceptions and faith, they will fit the one ultimate path—yours. Fundamentally, whether the faith you choose has a higher power that is around you or above you, or you believe that god, guru and self are all one and divinity is within you and that we are all intrinsically connected at every level of life, to practise a good hustle you need to simply have a trust in your self. You also need a motivation to do your work with the intention of unconditional love and selfless service that is vastly bigger and more compelling than simply bringing home a wage and acquiring more stuff. As far as God goes, you get to choose your own terminology here. My stance on G/god as a word softened and shifted when I came to understand god/s via exposure to Hinduism and interpretations of Buddhism. These traditions see god as something within. It was nothing short of a revelation that divinity and enlightenment were something that I had responsibility for and, more critically, control over, through my actions but most importantly through my mind. I'm assuming here that you aren't Richard Dawkins or Friedrich Nietzsche. That you have bought, borrowed or pirated a copy of *The Good Hustle* because you already subscribe to the idea that there is more than just each of us, separate and alone, returning to carbon at the end of life. Let's agree, then, that we all come to the party with a faith of some sort.

With that groundwork laid out, you will have your own way of describing what your faith is and how you experience it. Your version of the divine is the only one that matters for you. It could simply be the feeling you get being in nature, riding a horse, or listening to the sea. It could be how you feel when you sit in meditation and find your breath for that one moment of clarity and stillness. Ultimately, it is the moment you lose yourself as you the doer, and become you, just being.

Indian yoga master B.K.S. Iyengar in *Light on Life* puts in perspective the way we tend to see divinity and spirituality as an 'acquisition'. He sees the very idea of a 'spiritual path' as a misnomer, that moving along a path towards divinity infers that it is outside of us, rather than being something that is, by definition, everywhere all the time. He suggests instead that if we clean and tidy our houses—body, mind and spirit—then we might one day notice that divinity has been sitting quietly waiting for us to notice it all along.

The *Frozen* Theme Song Principle

The second thematic stream throughout *The Good Hustle* that I want to put some context around is surrender. Surrender in the Western usage is seen as defeat or collapse, rather than a relinquishing of control. In the Yoga Sutras, Patanjali transforms 'surrender' from this sort of last-resort, emergency response into an essential ongoing practice. But who or what are we surrendering to, how do we do it, and why is it so important?

In the yogic canon, surrender is to a higher power, to a union with the divine. Surrender shifts our perspective from the obsession with 'I'—our narrow individual concerns and perspective that cause so much of the mind's distraction and create a sense of separation from who we are, and how we connect with everything and everyone.

Since surrender focuses not on ego but on dissolving ourselves into a universal consciousness, it reunites us with our true self. This is a massive concept, the understanding of both our innate truth and self, which is a lifetime's undertaking. By way of shorthand, I am using it in the context of being closer to an understanding of the essence of who we are, how to make sense of that and how we can apply it to our daily lives. Surrender is not an intellectual understanding, it is a true physical and mindful relinquishing of all control.

If you were to think about it in the way people often describe watershed moments in their lives, they use phrases like hitting 'rock bottom'—when they have no other solution but to turn everything over to whatever higher power they are calling out to. As the wartime saying goes, there are no atheists in the trenches. There is nothing left but faith and hope that someone, or something, somewhere will intervene. It's the step after overwhelmed when we realise we simply can't do it all. Surrender for many of us comes initially from crisis, or, as author and yogi Ahimsa

Saraswati puts it, 'Most of us need a massive pummelling before we give up on being the doer. Not easy and deeply humbling.'

A footnote on surrender: if you are wondering about the actual process, it is not so much an action as a practice. You need to surrender over and over, to consciously release your tight grip on everything all the time. Entrepreneurs are often guilty of holding on to their ideas with all their might, of feeling they are the sole captain sailing the ship, with full responsibility for everything. Nun-uh. If you really want to let your ideas fly, you need to be collaborative. You need to give it up, and ask for support, to turn it all over to something, someone, somewhere and simply trust. The act of surrender is coupled with the act of asking for help, acknowledging that you are gently and graciously allowing others to be part of your journey. This is a deliciously long lifetime process, which forces you right back into the moment, as you can't see the short-, medium- and long-term outcomes. You can certainly be clear on what you would like them to be, and put yourself in the way of opportunity, but you also need the secret sauce that flavours all successful entrepreneurs—agility. You need to be available for whatever shows up for you. If it looks like the polar opposite of what you had dialled up in your wish list of life, you need to be ready to greet the situation like a beloved family member and open the door to the experience, without clinging to the imaginary future experience you had already created in your mind. As Elsa would say, 'Let it go.'

Unconditional Love (Conditions Apply)

Okay, we're only at the beginning here and I don't want you freaking out that you don't know your asana from your divine. Suffice to say, we have our definitions and context for the bigger questions without answers, and you know what the intentions behind the use of these words are. But wait. There is one more. And it's a biggie. Yoga is a devotional business. It asks you to surrender to a love that is universal, an unconditional love, and this is the third definition we need to explore, probably with some caution.

Perhaps you don't even have a sense of what unconditional love is. Many of us don't, having mainly been raised in relationships with parents and family in a Western culture where love is largely transactional. It might have looked something like this scenario: if you behave in the supermarket, you'll be rewarded with love and a chocolate bar, if you scream the aisles down, you will be scolded, shamed and have love withheld. The classic binary of good and bad, love not love, sugar given or withheld.

Of course the majority of mothers understand the unconditional love equation and what they would instantly and instinctively do to ensure the safety and wellbeing of their child as different from the well-worn path to stop-the-supermarket-screaming scenario. But that is not so transparent, well understood, or as regularly articulated as love being a reward as part of an overt exchange. Most kids aren't being raised to know intrinsically that they are complete and perfect as they are in their experience of this life. That all they need to do is go out into the world with curiosity and wonder, and trust that their life will be played out as intended, as they grow through failure and learning. If that were the message, our systems of education and interactions with each other would be entirely different. And not in a bad way. We would have a world peopled with well-adjusted, loving beings who cared deeply for the welfare of their fellow humans.

But we don't.

We have continents populated by people frantically searching for their Passion, desperately seeking to get off the endless cycle of work and material reward without basic happiness and peace; caught in their own private pain, anxiety and isolation, desperate for external love and approval. The Western world is built on transactions and material rewards, so little wonder that this is how we model our relationships. Unconditional love is what we aspire to in romantic love—which is what we think unconditional love is or should be. I subscribe to the idea that romantic love, as grand and swoony as it is, is entirely conditional. We enter relationships with an idea of what we are getting and giving to our partner; all good relationships are a series of mutually negotiated exchanges. Doesn't sound quite as Hallmark when described this way, does it? I'm not suggesting that the love in relationships isn't genuine and deep, but I hazard it isn't unconditional—and nor should it be. We all need to have boundaries and standards of behaviour we accept and don't accept in our interpersonal relationships, especially our intimate ones.

If we work off the 'I will always love you' Whitney Houston song sheet (or Dolly Parton's, if the original is more your speed), with the inference that love will be given no matter what happens, things can go kinda pear-shaped. A scenario sadly played out in Whitney's own life and tragic end. Just to reinforce, conditional love isn't bad, it is the reality of human-to-human relationships. The rules of unconditional love are, of course, that there are no rules as the love is unconditional. You simply surrender to your higher power, or god or guru or spirit or self-belief, or whom or whatever you have decided embodies the feeling of embracing the beloved for you. That surrender is in the knowledge that you are going to receive complete and total unconditional love. For everything past, present and future, without judgement or criticism, just pure acceptance. You are loved exactly and explicitly as you are in this moment. No matter what. In return, you accept that everything in your life is a direct result of your surrender, and is part of your journey, of your dharma, and is within that unfolding grace. Everything, even the shameful stuff that you would put in the not-so-good box is a necessary part of your evolution to enlightenment, or wherever you've set your coordinates to go. In Buddhism this is your karma ripening. Take a breath. This concept is massive.

Acceptance, surrender, unconditional: all notions that ask for a large—actually, a total—lack of control. As we all break into a cold sweat, I acknowledge this brutally challenges the Western mindset. We have to give over the reins of our mind controlling us with continual reactive thoughts. And not just give them over, but intellectually relinquish control and trust to the somewhat intangible idea of 'being in the moment'. This is a big leap. The biggest. And we aren't always rewarded in a direct and instantly gratifying way. So we have given up control and have to commit to the long haul, with no surety that what we think the benefits will be are going to appear. There's no road map and nothing except faith in the divine to be our GPS. Feel free to exit here. But if you are prepared to consider the opportunities, detangling these ideas from our everyday way of living and recontextualising them into livin' la yogi loca, the proposition begins to make more sense.

When we surrender in the yogic sense, we give ourselves fully, in the spirit of unconditional love. There aren't reciprocal conditions, in that we don't give ourselves in love so we can wildly manifest money, houses and dreamboat partners. We don't give ourselves in love to nice people and not to the ones we don't like the look of. When we are all one, we are *all one*. Even with your ex and your asshole boss. All of the activities of our lives become part of our yoga practice. It can exist in every action and interaction, through a conscious dedication to oneness with others, and a determination to keep the mind clear and present in the now. This can be a game changer when it comes to mundane, everyday chores, as it makes these ordinary acts offerings of unconditional love. This view of unconditional love and its enormity takes a while to infuse; and it will be an ongoing theme of the book. While you are turning it over in your mind, let us return to some ancient wisdoms and the context in which we start the journey to adopting this mindset into our lives and business practices.

Bigger Magic

In her excellent book *Big Magic*, Elizabeth Gilbert recounts reading a blog post by writer Mark Manson (he of *The Subtle Art of Not Giving a F*ck*) that said the secret to finding your purpose in life was to answer the one big question: 'What is your favourite flavour of shit sandwich?' It's a crude analogy for what is an often unspoken truth—every pursuit in life comes with some unpalatable side effects, no matter how much Passion and Purpose sauce you've ladled on. Zen Buddhism gives us another version of this: 'Before enlightenment chop wood, carry water. After enlightenment, chop wood, carry water.' This saying can be interpreted in a number of ways with regard to the cyclical nature of life and death and the continual process of learning. However, I think it also fits into the spirit of *The Good Hustle*. When all actions and activities are being done with the intention of love and service to others without seeking personal acknowledgement or reward, it doesn't matter what you are doing. It all has the same intrinsic feeling of love—even the shit-sandwich-flavoured bits.

Not seeking personal benefits as your main priority doesn't mean there won't be benefits. It just won't be a reward that comes like a massive sugar rush to your ego. Elevating you with uncontrollable endorphins only to drop you like a stone in the comedown and leave you tired, hungry and craving for more. The reward isn't external, or given to you. The reward is the practice. At first it will be an uncomfortable practice, as our mindset is geared towards work being personal, business being personal.

We are the doers, doing that thing that brings us money to conduct our transactional lives based on consumption, inputs and outputs. It's what brings us fame or personal recognition for our singular, spectacular endeavours. It is hard to imagine making the effort required to achieve anything if some personal, tangible reward isn't the carrot we are pursuing.

It is also hard to give up the drama.

We may think we aspire to being free of suffering, achieving liberation from our ordinary human unhappiness, released from the yoke of neurosis. But do we really? Suffering, in many cases, writes the narrative of our lives and provides a comfortable refuge from which to disengage our willpower muscles or our self-discipline. Of course that bad day at work means you need chocolate for comfort. Reminding yourself it is merely the human condition and getting on with life isn't nearly so sweet. It allows us to continue feeding the hungry ghosts that are our attachments. While it might seem counterintuitive, we are often a little bit, or a lot, in love with misery. If you're thinking 'That's crazy talk', then ask yourself why aren't you already liberated from suffering, happy and free with a spacious mind? The formula has been publicly available for centuries.

The answer is: it is hard, requires discipline and dedication, and it is not a quick fix. A cocktail is a quick fix; a block of chocolate is a quick fix, turning off the alarm and rolling over instead of going to the gym is a quick fix; and all come with a little gratification buzz, which nicely distracts us for a moment. That you are even reading this book, however, infers that you are ready to get off this diet made up of tiny bites and sips of suffering, and chow down on the high-fibre daily goodness of a practice that will ultimately make you feel better, even if it is a little unpalatable at first. We all have the capacity to concentrate on a single matter at hand when we are engrossed in doing something we love. That is the grit and resilience spoken about in growth mindset. The challenge is preparing your mind to release its love affair with the spectacular allure of sense gratifications. You need to focus on stilling down. On becoming clear and attaining the discipline needed for focus, in a culture of attention-grabbing distractions. This is made harder by the fact that it is achieved through mastering tough and not particularly fascinating exercises, such as observing the breath or sitting meditating with a straight spine. Practising the ideas contained in the eight limbs of yoga so you can know your mind is real, as the mind is the root from which all of our action and reaction happen. In this context, it is worth taking the time to get intimate with your most powerful tool.

Mind Over Matter

You cannot do yoga.
Yoga is your natural state.

SHARON GANNON, YOGI, ACTIVIST AND
FOUNDER OF JIVAMUKTI YOGA

Knowing your mind is a lifetime process. It is the relinquishing of the belief that the world is happening outside of you, that you are not central to all events and happenings, that you don't somehow control your engagement with the world. There are undoubtedly things that you perceive you don't control—trivia like the weather, non-trivia like major disasters. What is a fact, however, is that we all control our re-action and our beliefs. I've split up the 're' from the action to underscore that the way we respond to situations is very much a chain of energy and behaviour. What action you witness, you 're' action; in other words, you interpret the behaviour through your own mind and creative narrative, and your actions follow. You choose this reaction, actively, although the habit of choosing it may well be unconscious if you've been re-acting in the same ways for a long time.

You might re-action a situation of drama and conflict by re-acting out that drama in response rather than just being an observer. You might action it on a deep, cellular level, taking your pain, hurt or shock internally, and mentally acting out all of the ways you could have or should have behaved and responded. Often in these situations where pain is internalised, you will have created a story about how to re-act, and treat in the same way every situation that reminds you of the preceding events. If each of us is a character in our own re-active narratives, very few of us are exercising the option to choose our own endings. It's a fixed mindset groundhog day and we are stuck in the loop of everything being preordained and done *to* us. We behave as though our narrative is being written by someone else, and we are in a continual flow of reaction and response. It is little wonder that so many of us are affected by anxiety and hypersensitivity, with our bodies in a perpetual fight-or-flight mode, waiting for the next page in the story to turn. We just don't realise we are actually holding the pen.

So, how to take back our stories and be our own directors in the film of our lives, without also being the perpetual internal armchair critics who give us zero out of five? The answer is in choosing to (firstly) make friends with, and then collaborate with, our minds. A purely discipline-based approach to stopping the lurching wave of emotion in all situations, and breathing into an empowered state of surrender. This is a choice that involves learning meditation and mindfulness techniques, being able to identify where you habitually re-act, and stop it. You need to understand your mind and thus your re-actions.

It's a simple premise, sure, but simple is not always easy. You are performing conditioned responses to situations, ones that you may, as an adult, have never questioned before. Your trigger is being tripped and you fire first, without aim. The power of the mind can be devastating, but it can also be astounding. If you can manage your mind, you can discover who you really are. As you will see when we get into breaking down the eight limbs of yoga against the stages of your new business or creative project, the mind management piece is ultimately the underpinning of your business management. The two aren't separate or separable.

Please Sir, Can I ~~Have~~ Enough?

It's interesting that when we talk about the stories that form our way of seeing and being, we infrequently mean positive stories. We almost exclusively build our identities on the ways we aren't enough, building a wall of failings rather than a pathway of successes. We are quick to catalogue a litany of things about ourselves that we don't love; they hang off us like invisible weights, heavy and restrictive of freely moving, thinking and being. The first steps in getting to a place where we can surrender and embrace unconditional love, where we can swim around in that salty buoyant sea, is to release the weights. To do this, we have to honestly investigate the roots of our stories, the emotional patterns that sit behind them, then release these as fiction so we can move on to living from fact. In Buddhism this would be termed moving from the unreal to the real—the unreal being samsara, where we are seduced by attachment to material goods and pleasure. The unreal is our belief that these things bring us happiness, and that they are permanent fixtures in our lives. The real is when we have polished the dust off the mirror of our true nature and can see clearly who we really are, and consequently are able to make choices and live our lives from a place of authenticity.

I've noticed one of the big impediments for women in getting their dreams up and running is the capacity to not be enough. Women seem particularly good at the amazing binary of simultaneously being excellent and never being good enough. It's one of our key multi-tasking achievements. I don't think I've ever met an intelligent, strong, beautiful, compassionate, successful woman (a category that covers all women) who, once you scratch the surface, isn't racked with the same deep fears and insecurities that seem to universally plague our gender. I have, however, met many men who believe with every cell of their being that they are truly, deeply, contentedly great.

This is not a him–her, Mars–Venus, war of the sexes argument; it is, however, truth-speaking regarding the way we as women manage to tease out our every last flaw and fear for the world to critique, when men in most cases are not similarly compelled to be so constantly self-excoriating. This has significant impacts when it comes to pursuing your business ideas. You need to be able to muster unshakeable belief when it comes to dealing with the many hurdles that will appear at the most inconvenient times. Insecurity needs to meet bravery and self-belief in the middle, and modify your reactions; managing your mind makes managing your decisions much simpler.

Meditation and yoga can transform your mind. By adopting a yogic lifestyle, the dust begins to be cleared from your self—but it is also a confronting process where long-held and buried parts have to reveal themselves to be processed and integrated. Therapy exists for this reason, and I totally subscribe to utilising professionals when needed to move the healing along when you feel stuck or unable to work the next bit out. Surrender was the key for me—I'd already invested plenty of time and money across years into trying to offload the feeling I wasn't where I was meant to be or 'living my Purpose', and I knew it was within me, not within my circumstance, that these negative and critical feelings and voices arose. It was clear I couldn't figure it out by myself, and so I literally surrendered to a variety of teachings, teachers and experiences to reveal the answers to me in their own perfect time.

Excavating the unreal to make way for the real is not a trivial exercise. Most of the patterns that have clouded the mirror of self begin in childhood, and by the time we have the vision to recognise them as actual impediments, they are well entrenched. The process of addressing the emotional patterns that have developed from childhood is very personal, and you have to work out what best suits your style of emotional and psychological investigation.

My patterns were so common, I simply believed I wasn't enough, and so nothing I ever did was okay. As well as not being enough, I was really afraid. I was afraid of what people thought of me, of people not liking me, of making the wrong decision, of failing, being criticised and ultimately abandoned by my tribe.

Fear Itself

Fear drove all my decision-making and re-actions. It was so intrinsic I didn't realise that it was in the driving seat, and I was somewhere in the boot of the car with duct tape over my mouth and cable ties round my wrists. My fear was completely out of proportion to the actual reality of my life. I was creating a cellular war zone and had been doing so since I was a child; no wonder things were getting so out of control in my mind and body with the accumulation of those four-lane fear highways I had built in my neural pathways. When you are coming from a place of fear, it is nigh on impossible to experience love and grace, to be agile and curious. The field of vision is so close to you that you are barely able to look up from your flight-or-fight path to see what is going on around you. When you do, everything is viewed through that lens of asking when the next crisis is coming and how you can combat it. It is an incredibly small radius to try to manufacture the capacity to love expansively and magnanimously. How do you feel connected to the world and all the people in it when you are hunkered down in a bomb shelter of flesh and bones?

My story is by no means unique. Early parental death pulled the rug from under me, and it took me a long time to regain my balance in trusting that what I loved and doted on wouldn't be taken away. In the pantheon of childhoods that set you up for this type of fear-based mindset, mine was nowhere near the razor wire in the spectrum of trauma some children experience. Without comparison to the unique experience of others, however, the commonness of my story is that many, many of us are living in these fear bubbles, getting along in the world to a greater or lesser degree, but completely restrained from our greatness by our not enoughness. We are unable to see and grasp our potential, and, more critically, unable to hear and access our true nature of selves. So everything that we do is based on a false perception of who we are and our capabilities—and consequently, we do what we think we should, not what we are destined to, in the hope of pleasing and being loved. The real love that is missing is, sadly, the love of ourselves.

The most terrifying thing about living a life based on fear is that we are simply existing for the external view and action of others. Fear-based existence is easy to get away with in a society where collectively this is our version of living. In our separateness and fear, we aren't alone. The stories that we tell each other in the twenty-four-hour news cycle, gossip cycle and social media cycle completely reinforce the rule of fear. It's like the new hero's journey is based on being born, being afraid, getting stuck, struggling and suffering, prolonging life while fearing death, and ultimately dying. It's finite, fixed and to a degree elite—you can have a higher quality of fear and suffering based on wealth and status, as you have so much more to lose. Fear robs us of being in the present. We are living in our minds in an unknown place and time, fighting battles that haven't started with adversaries who don't exist.

20/20 Faith

So how does fear link to starting your good hustle? To surrender to unconditional love, to let go of our attachments and cravings, and live from that vulnerable space of openness, there has to be trust. Complete trust. The kind of trust that allows you to be blindfolded and led by the hand knowing you won't come to any harm. Perhaps this is the root of the expression 'blind faith'. You have to see and experience your own divinity within all of the reality of your perceived flaws and failings, and in doing so, you also have to see everyone else's. Buddhist nun Tenzin Palmo believes that faith is an expression of courage, not a kind of blindness or belief in something just because you are credulous. In handing over control you accept a trip without any kind of clear destination, but it is a journey full of the daily pleasure of living—without fear. Exchanging self for others is not a situation where one is lost or traded for the other, leaving a deficit. Adopting the service of others in the mode of goodness gives us inner courage, with which we can bravely step into the most difficult of situations.

It is unsurprising that Tenzin Palmo holds that belief. She has an extraordinary story—at a young age, in the early 1960s, she was called to find a faith. She eventually dedicated herself to Buddhism and finding enlightenment, setting off from England to India on a freight ship to meet her lama. As part of her practice she entered a remote cave in the high Himalayas and stayed there in meditation for twelve years. On her return to the world, she began spreading the dharma through her teaching and writing, and champions tirelessly for funding the nunnery she has built in India.

In interviews it is often suggested to Tenzin that being in the cave was easier than trying to practise mind management in the chaos and stress of the West. She utterly refutes that, and points out that in a cave there are no distractions from the self. The removal of distractions, pleasure and noise means facing the experience of our minds and selves directly. This opens us to the possibility of recognising that whatever we experience—love, loneliness, hate, jealousy, joy, greed—is, in essence, an expression of the fundamentally unlimited potential of our awakened nature. When we have this awareness, there are no more surprises within to react to. It is not an easy awakening.

This concept doesn't imply there is nothing to fear. Instead it entreats you to change your relationship to re-action through control of the mind. In your process of surrender, you are accepting that what happens next, or what happens now, is exactly what is meant to happen, and it is how you interpret it and react that determines the experience you have of it. The limiting ideas we hold about ourselves, others, and every other experience can be unlearned. In that moment, suffering ends. There is nothing to fear, nothing to resist. Not even death can trouble you. The Dalai Lama describes Westerners' lives as simply lurching away from any kind of pain or suffering and compulsively leaning in to pleasure. This is the reality of re-action, that we are ruled by sense experiences and our likes and dislikes, as though each experience is going to be a lasting and permanent state. We don't have the mental discipline to stay in the centre and note the feeling without drama, accepting that this is what is now, not what will always be. This concept works in lock step with your karma and dharma, presupposing that you are viewing this life as a carryover from the last, on the long middle road to liberation and enlightenment.

PART TWO

DESPERATELY SEEKING DHARMA

Find out who you are and do it on purpose.

DOLLY PARTON, SINGER, SONGWRITER, ACTOR,
BUSINESSWOMAN ... LIVING LEGEND

WHEN YOU PINPOINT HAPPINESS ARISING,
ASK YOURSELF WHAT IS HAPPENING
IN THIS MOMENT WHEN YOU FIND YOU
ARE LOVING WHAT YOU ARE DOING.
THIS IS THE POINT ON THE CHART WHERE
YOU DROP A PIN, A DEFINITE CLUE TO YOUR
OWN HAPPY MAP.

What the Dharma?

You may wonder why dharma is so important in our discussions of getting your good hustle in order. Dharma, depending on your school of thought or religious lineage, can mean different things. In yoga, your dharma is what is right for you, it is the expression of your true self, so when you live your dharma things flow and you feel right in your own skin. The Hindu connotation is that your dharma is the right way to live. It's personal, in as much as only you are able to determine what your dharma is and, like a fingerprint, it is different for everyone. Some of us are born with a very clear sense of what we are here to do. I can only speculate on why that is, and, regardless, knowing it and living it doesn't always correlate. As discussed earlier, discovering your dharma can be a torturous process. It was for me, and I'm grateful in a schadenfreude kind of way that I share this torture with many millions of others. What does seem to be universal is that no matter how we try to navigate around it, or avoid it, we end up where we are meant to be, doing what we are meant to be doing. This is our dharma, and thus our right way to live. In being the right way to live, this notion is directly connected in Hinduism and Buddhism with karma.

Karma is simply translated as cause and effect. It is constant and perpetual and thus works in lock step with your dharma—as it is in the interests of minimising the action and (negative) re-action that you live mindfully in the right way. Living the right way means accumulating as little negative karma as possible, by living within the precepts of a yogic lifestyle. Karma in the West is often interpreted as a dramatic and instant retribution, like a bolt of lightning out of the blue striking down the errant offender. The Buddha says that karma is intention, that what we sow through our actions is not in fact measured by the doing of the action, but by the intention that sits behind it.

Accidentally pocketing someone's pen and discovering it when you get home isn't an act of theft, for example. Coveting the pen and strategically slipping it into your bag while the owner isn't looking, while feeling smug at your deception—that is theft. The intention is clearly different, as are the karmic outcomes. Far from being dramatic and showy, karma rightly understood is about our own responsibility for the transaction of action and intent from our minds. We are always making a choice in every micro action, and this is why control over the mind and a grasp on awareness is so critical to remaining in a place of loving kindness towards everything and everyone.

Unlike karma, there is in reality no simple English translation of dharma, and in the Buddhist traditions it means a subtly different thing. The Buddha taught a method of dharma or dharma practice, rather than a religion. The dharma in Buddhism, or Buddhadharma, is not something to believe in, but something to do. The Buddha challenged people to understand the nature of anguish/suffering, let go of its origins, realise its cessation, and bring into being a way of life that had at its heart the best interest of all sentient beings. The dharma is a method to be investigated and tried out. It starts by facing up to the universality of suffering, then proceeds to apply a set of practices to understand the human dilemma and work towards a resolution. Stay tuned for a deeper discussion of these ideas in the following chapters.

In a world where we are so influenced by the opinions and actions of others, and forensically study the minutiae of our lives through social media, our own dharma path is difficult to discern. When we live in a state of comparison and judgement, under the perpetual threat of criticism and social shaming, we end up parroting the behaviour of others, hoping that it will serve us and keep us under the radar. We do as we are told, or as we think we should, and hope that through this strategy happiness will appear. What we get from this is suffering and endless layers of false perceptions to reverse as we sink more deeply into the mire of sense attachments. In the process, getting further and further away from any possibility of resting comfortably in our own divinity. The purpose of dharma is not only to attain a union of the consciousness with the divine, it also suggests a code of conduct that is intended to secure worldly joys and supreme happiness. Adherents to this yogic way of thinking understand the attainment of the highest ideal and eternal bliss happens here and now on earth, and not somewhere in a place of separateness at death.

Escaping fear, embracing unconditional love, surrendering to divinity, and releasing yourself from the endless stories that define and narrate your experience are the goals of mind management, to get you to a place where you clearly know what your heart desires. But it is a practice. I've said it once and it will be oft repeated. Awareness of patterns and reactions doesn't make them simply disappear. As the meme tells us, one does not simply stop being enslaved to one's suffering. Suffering is, the Buddha would argue, what makes us human. It's not so much a negative thing as a thing, and our engagement with suffering and its myriad causes is the definition of humanness. Suffering is part of the pathway to surrender. When we don't try to stop it, but simply recognise it is going to be a feature of our existence, we take from it the power to throw us into the whirlpool of our minds.

Dharma Chameleon

Getting down to your good hustle, the clearing of patterns, the neutralising of fear, the revelation of what our individual right way to live might be, gives clarity to our purpose. So to begin the process of how this can connect with what we want to do, let's play a new version of that well-worn game 'What would you do if money was no object?' There is a flaw in that premise, so often used to help people get to the heart of what motivates them, as it assumes that money, and the acquisition of money, is the meta-motivator. A better way of framing the question is 'What makes you feel love?' No need to link it to financial gains or fancy career titles, as all of that is irrelevant if your work is a good hustle that comes from a place of love and devotion.

Many books and workshops on how to make a life you love, grow the business of your dreams and all the other marketing spin, need you to know where you want to go to get where you are going. But sometimes that isn't a reality—we simply don't know. We have to feel our way around in the dark a bit. The keyword is that we feel, and we develop those powers of intuition and our own internal compass to lead us to the twinkling lights of our magnificent dharma.

If I was to base this investigation on my own list of diverse childhood career aspirations, the common thread was that they were jobs that were of personal service to others in one way or another. The drive in me even at a really young age was to touch people's lives and offer some kind of loving support (literally, in the case of my prostitution aspirations). Writing also featured in what I wanted to do, and has continued to be an integral part of my life, work, study and growth. But writing isn't my dharma. It is an instrument of my dharma, which is actually teaching. Writing is a super form of expression, but in and of itself is a solo and removed activity, just me and my laptop and not a sentient being in sight.

The discovery of my dharma was the feeling I got when I saw people connect with their own purpose. It was in my entrepreneurship teaching and business development consultancy work—I was lit up inside by sharing with clients the moment that the dream they had kept away from the light, fearful of failure or defeated by their perceived limitations, could be a reality. When I help people through teaching them about how to merge sustainable business models with their own spiritual path, it gives me a particular feeling where I connect to a joy that is vast and contagious. Teaching for me isn't about having the knowledge, or even being the teacher. I don't have any sense of ownership. I see myself as an usher; I shine my torch on information that is unseen in the darkness. Different people need to see different things—I show them how to switch their own light on, then move on to the next project. The building, operating and executing is all down to the individual. This is a factor that I need to keep reminding myself of. Far more evolved people than I have been sucked in to the belief that they have a special gift only they can deliver (so not growth mindset). You know what they say—don't believe the hype. When you work in service or to be of benefit, the other person always comes first.

Mind Your Own Business

Everything begins in the mind, as only our perceptions define what is happening around us. You begin in the mind, business begins in the mind. Mind in the yogic understanding is both physical and subtle, and covers the entire body from the brain and nervous systems, spanning out to all of our sense organs, and our gross body which it controls and drives like a supercomputer. So much of the work of new business concepts happens in the mind before a Gantt chart is constructed, a Facebook page initiated or a dollar raised. Yet so little attention seems to be given to strengthening and managing the mind in discussions of entrepreneurship and ideation.

To rock a good hustle, however, the mind is the first port of call in establishing the right attitude and capability to step out of our striving and non-thriving into our business or creative practice. It is never too soon to work on stilling the churning waters of the mind, and prepare a calm work surface. We don't need any new tools, we can start with what we have right now. By understanding our mind, everything is transformed. And like charity, transformation begins at home and must be started by you.

Ultimately, surrendering what we cannot control allows the ego to relax and lose the anxiety of is own infinitesimally small self in the expanse of interconnection with others. It is timely here to investigate the ego and what it really means. So often we use a concept or have a superficial understanding of what something means through the collective use of a term. The ego is one such term, and is bandied about in a way that infers it is some kind of dark controller of your personality over which you have no personal agency. We can't, contrary to popular belief, just let go of the ego. That's like letting go of an arm. It is part of us, and a necessary part.

From the Western psychological perspective, the ego is akin to a physical entity, and represents the personality, the 'I' of a person, the beliefs underpinning what and who we are. The ego is difficult to see, because it hides behind opinions that appear true—our attachment to descriptions of our identity—and because we haven't practised looking. One of the most deceptive aspects of the ego is that it generates powerful emotional reactions, and then blames us for how it made us feel. All of which leaves us at the mercy of the ego, and removes our own capacity to manage our emotional states and swings. This is where the management of the mind is so critical, as nothing really exists outside of us, and therefore all states are within and in our control.

Sure, there is no denying that there are external events and triggers that act as catalysts for us to make a choice on how we react. A mind that is regularly interrogated through meditation and mindfulness takes on the events perceived as good and those perceived as bad with equal curiosity. To investigate the totality of your being, the negative and the positive are equal partners in how we perceive ourselves—of course, too often with a strong emphasis on the negative. Instead, see the ego as your agitated, uncontrolled mind, apportioning blame and playing the victim. By using meditation and turning within, observing your mental state without attaching emotion to it, all situations are understandable and can be released with a loose grip, rather than dwelled upon. In this way the ego is assimilated as part of us, and becomes a collaborator and communicator of our inner state, a tool for awareness rather than a despotic ruler.

So what can the ego communicate to us? The reaction of emotion is one of the most obvious ways that we know our mind is in sway and ego is acting out. It is this swing of the pendulum that is a giant distraction from being present. Working in mindfulness in cahoots with the ego when an emotion arises, rather than in re-action, allows us to see that emotion from the standpoint of a loving, compassionate observer. The key here is observing its arising, and its origins—what situation was the precursor? When it is revealed what our reactive patterns are, this is the area we can focus on to start digging, removing the shadows, and in time clearing out the rubbish from our mind and our heart.

A metaphor for this work is that of hard, exhausting physical labour—the excavation and patience required by prospecting, where it can take hours to only scratch the surface of ground buried by years of build-up. And patience is a vital attribute in mastery of the mind. Nothing is achieved in a rush. Patience, paired with disciplined practice, brings with it the required willpower to stay in it for the long game. Got grit? When you adopt the practice of the yogi, you know how short a lifetime is, and how many are potentially required to get stuff done. In time there is no willpower required—you want to do it all the time, as without the practice, life is empty. Of course, this is also exactly the new groove that we want in your neural neighbourhood for the work required to create your business. Our goal in the preparatory phase is then to be content to work consistently towards our own authenticity—that moment of clarity when we feel on the path to dharma.

Nothing is Everything, Everything is Nothing

Along with the Yoga Sutras, the teachings that underpin the massively broad church that is Buddhism have some concepts that are a very useful contribution to training our minds, and preparing ourselves for approaching business from the perspective of it being a good hustle. Buddhist teachings essentially tell us that suffering exists, and thus ending suffering for all sentient beings is of primary importance. Buddhism also teaches impermanence, and that nothing has an intrinsic existence of its own, including ourselves and our identities.

Everything comes into being because of causes and conditions, so things only exist because of their interdependence on other things. Buddhists see these interdependencies as part of the fundamental existence of everything, and by taking on these ideas, it is very hard to feel separate, isolated or alone. You can take a look at *anything* and break it down to its causes and conditions. Confused? Let's clarify with an example. Imagine a cake: we think of a cake as a solid thing that exists. You've eaten a cake (um, many), you know that a cake is real and three dimensional, and yet a cake does not exist as an intrinsic thing—it only exists as the culmination of all the things that make it a cake: eggs, flour, sugar, fats, air, heat, a greased tin and its other ingredients. A cake isn't independently existent, it's made of components. And so is everything else. You can deconstruct anything and come to the same conclusion; things only come into being as a result of their causes and conditions, and the causes and conditions have their own causes and conditions, and this goes on and on and on. The Twitter version of this is that everything is interconnected and nothing exists—including us humans, without the dependencies that arise from causes and conditions. It is an epic mind-bending consideration, but one that, when firmly entrenched in the brain, is strangely freeing and comforting.

Everything about us is in constant change, from the trillions of cells that make up our body, to the multitude of processes that create thoughts, emotions, reactions, opinions and beliefs. We are not us, we are a collective of cells, atoms, water, calcium, however you want to break us down biologically. We are not static objects, we are works in progress, with mind-boggling, complex processes happening 24/7 that all depend on each other. Thich Nhat Hanh, a Vietnamese Buddhist monk, author and peace activist, calls this state 'interbeing'. This term embraces the sense of compassion and love that comes from connection. Because all things are interdependent and in a constant state of change, all things must also be impermanent.

When we adopt the view that everything is impermanent, we are released (in theory at least) from attachment and, in this school of thought, from the suffering that comes with striving to hold on to something that is not going to be around forever, or the sorrow that comes with loss. If we behave in the mode of impermanence, it pushes us to be in the moment, to appreciate what we have in the now. It forces us to accept the peace that comes with knowing that if everything is constantly changing, there will never be a void when something leaves. Cause and condition will always instantly find a set of elements to replace it with. The problem is that we know this and yet we continue to cling to things as if they were permanent, because we want these things to last (at least during our lifetime). That doesn't mean it's easy when we lose something or someone that is precious, it just means that the recovery from suffering is able to be understood at a heart and mind level when we learn to see things as they really are—impermanent.

The Two I's

Impermanence and interdependence in business is a good thing: here's how and why. Part of the difficulty for many people in starting up a new business or bringing their ideas to market is that there is a fixed idea of what they are providing, the pathway that will get them there, and the customer whose problem they are solving with their (and by 'their' I mean 'your') genius. None of this is wrong, and traditional approaches to business planning focus strongly on having these elements and answers in place prior to market entry. You are meant to have risk managed all of the potential problems you can think of, troubleshot like an Olympic marksman, and largely eliminated any obstacle likely to get in your path. This is all well and good if you are in possession of the entire spectrum of causes and conditions. Which, of course, none of us are. Once we hit the market and unanticipated things start coming at us right and left, we default to that next setting on the entrepreneur dial: flowing around problems. We are still trying to fix the issue to get to the original destination. When we flow around something, we still head in approximately the same direction, with a mildly altered route.

When seeing your emerging business from the viewpoint of the two I's—interdependence and impermanence—you can be radically agile with no suffering. You can accept when things need to do a 180-degree turnaround, and not have a moment of clinging to the idea of what might have been. Your only relationship is to what is, and the causes and conditions that constitute your market entry in the moment. In the early stages of coming up with an idea for a new business, project or venture, the process of refining your idea is a straightforward formula. You see a gap in the market, a problem to be solved, and you have an elegant solution to that problem that meets the market at a point where the cost of solving the problem is acceptable to the customer and delivers surplus revenue. While this follows a relatively linear path, it is always iterative. The place you start is rarely where you finish, especially if you are using lean start-up practices, where the minimum viable product (MVP) is what goes to market, and interactivity with your clients drives the development into a third space of creativity and evolution between the idea and the end user. This thinking, pioneered by Eric Reis in his book *The Lean Startup*, was a shift from previous thinking, whereby companies completely developed a product prior to release in the market. The practice came from the tech and digital sector as it made sense to be able to release several versions of software, apps and the like, and use the collective wisdom of the customer to enhance the product rather than making the assumption that the creators and developers had all the answers.

The lean start-up was more than a process innovation for launching your business on a shoestring, it started a new conversation about user or customer agency and the power of collaboration. Knowledge and its power became democratised and, more interestingly, consumers became collaborators and in doing so had a much deeper connection with a brand when they had a say in the creation of products and services. They weren't being dictated to anymore, they were being asked their opinion, and rewarded with products that were functional and affordable. Sure, this is trickier to pull off with a mass-produced item like a car. But more and more cars are about customisation, and it may do excellent things for struggling traditional industries if they did more MVPs and fewer top-down sales.

We will look at how to make an MVP and what type could suit your business later in the book, so for now just understand this as going to market with an early working prototype. The link here is that everyone knows the MVP stage is just the beginning. It is absolutely, unequivocally impermanent. There are plenty of leaps of faith in this process.

When the lean method came out initially, it flipped the usual practice of having a complete product enter the market. The big shift was the realisation that you can't always anticipate fully what the market actually needs unless you have a conversation with your end users first. You can see a problem that needs solving and come up with a creative solution, but you and your team, if you have one, are a very limited number of thinkers. By reaching out and releasing an MVP, you are surrendering to the market. You are surrendering to hundreds, thousands or millions of people who can engage with your idea, give you feedback and make it better. You don't know the outcome, and you don't need to, as in theory the best outcome will be the one that emerges through the collaborative journey.

By just looking at the parallels between this approach to a new product or service, and the approach to our lives of working in the yogic way, you can see how the elements harmonise. This message will be sounded loud and clear in as many ways as possible. Surrender. You don't have to know everything, you don't have to do everything. You just have to be alert and listen to the strong voice, feeling or desire that niggles at you and tells you that there is a role for you to play in bringing an idea into the world. Get used to change and see it as a constant positive. Call it agility. Train yourself to operate this way by knowing yourself and your mind intimately.

I think that often when we have this calling to contribute a new business idea, a concept for a good hustle, the default position is to reject it, to say no. If we aren't enough in our everyday life, how can we possibly rearrange the pieces of our lives to enable something as big as a new business to get out of our heads and into the world? It's a fair question; especially if you haven't got any experience in business, or have very specific areas of expertise. Even more so if you have no idea how you would fund your idea, or where the time to do all of this would come from. You can see how it's pretty easy to slam the door shut in the face of opportunity. Based on everything we think we know about our limitations, our can'ts and don'ts, and the overwhelming sea of anxiety that can accompany pursuing an idea, it is amazing that anyone ever actions their big ideas. But they do, and usually because the voice of urgency to get it done is louder than the voice of resistance. Being able to hear the voice of urgency is easier once the mind is quiet and the body still, which is one of the many gifts a meditation practice will bring.

From Side Hustle to Good Hustle

The good hustle pre-training is where the heavy lifting gets done, as once the game has started, you have to rely on your newly minted neural pathways to react with a loose grip and a steady trust in the now. This can be of some comfort if you are straining like a greyhound at the gate to race your idea to market but are held back by the regular impediments that life throws your way, especially when work, family and children are involved. Delays are a convenient time to do more practice, on the mat and the meditation cushion. It is also an opportunity to engage in further conversations with potential customers and collaborators.

Building an awareness of your key skill sets allows you to get started pointing in the right direction. If we backtrack to the question 'What is it that makes you feel love?', this is usually where there is a confluence of skill mastery and motivation. You can make a list, and it may be at this point that you recognise your existing work bears very little relationship to that which makes you burst with love. Don't even try to link your list to your existing work if that becomes a blockage to getting familiar with your joy. For some readers, you may well feel that all of your work is repellent and represents a series of millstones rather than milestones in your life. No matter. There will be moments where you hook in to that feeling of absorption and joy, where the world is going by and you are in the flow with it.

It could be when you are making coffee for your co-workers, or counselling the CFO on their unhappy marriage. It could be when you are arranging some flowers for the front desk or creating systems in messy digital files. Be forensic in your investigations and don't dismiss a current situation. When you pinpoint happiness arising, ask yourself what is happening in this moment when you find you are loving what you are doing. This is the point on the chart where you drop a pin, a definite clue to your own happy map.

Keep investigating what gets your joy going. Give this exercise some time and oxygen, it isn't a tick-and-flick operation. Remember the virtue of patience and cultivate it here, along with self-kindness. If you're imagining everyone else gets the answer straight away, they don't and your own experience is incomparable anyway. So take it slowly and lovingly. You may need to physically stop reading this book and get still, settle into a comfortable pose or seated in a quiet place where you can have some time to just be alone and undisturbed. Close your eyes and try to conjure up images of activities and moments in your life where you have felt a deep sense of love and connection, where you have been truly happy, or even just content—a much underrated state of being. Of course you also don't know what is outside of your own experience either, which means that feeling is often a better guide than something you can put a label on.

Just a note about confusing these feelings of love and happiness with attachment to sensory pleasure—if a recurring vision of your happy place is smashing down a bucket of ice cream, this may not be happiness but numbing unhappiness and discomfort through sense indulgence. Logically, this is not an activity that you would do over a longer period of time to gain mastery over your mind, become an entrepreneur and spread the devotion. Unless your name was Ben or Jerry.

Keep looking for signs of happiness. Keep noting feelings of contentment. Become aware of their timing and correlations. These are signals for you to help you on your path. When you have these happy signals in sufficient quantity to feel they are a representative sample of your true self, the next step is to cast around for an opportunity that could be big enough to scale into a business for you.

Look from every imaginable angle, and even then remain open to more. Our humanness has blinkers that leave us with very narrow vision. Remember, as B.K.S. Iyengar says, what you are looking for is already quietly within, waiting for the mess and chaos of your mind to calm, the dust to settle, to be revealed. Don't get frustrated if you don't get immediate answers. Always keep in mind that you are taking on a practice; this is a long game, the longest. It's the game of your life.

Aside from these signs, there are some other indicators that you have found your good hustle dharma mojo, and are on the way to living in flow and turning self-love into selfless service. Once your idea has settled and taken shape, you can apply the following four questions—which I call the Good Hustle Hurdles—to it and tune in to your inner compass for guidance:

1. Will you enjoy doing it?
2. Does it come easily?
3. Does it give benefits to others?
4. Can you see yourself doing it for a long time?

The Good Hustle Hurdles

If I was to apply these questions to my next venture of teaching good hustle workshops around the globe, here is what it might look like.

1. Will You Enjoy It?

If you think about what you are intending to do, can you project that joy and happiness onto every conceivable part of it (keeping the blinker limitations and shit sandwich parts in mind)? When running workshops, there are a lot of logistics, a lot of marketing and promotion, and work to remove any barriers to participation for potential clients. There is also a fair amount of administrivia and detail, some of which is definitely a filling in my shit sandwich! Most of this is easily manageable with good assistance and taking advantage of great virtual assistants (VAs) and project management software. Happily, this is a minor part of the real joy: working with inspiring people and watching them transform into good hustlers full of joy and meaning and making a difference. I can tick that one off.

2. Does It Come Easily?

To be working in your own flow—though you can always continue to develop—the basic skills required and delivery of the idea have to come easily. This means if you want to be an engineer, you will need to have a love for maths and physics and have completed a degree in engineering before you can begin. If you want to run a doggy day care, you will need to love animals, have an affinity for communicating with them, a willingness to clean up a lot of poop and a large, secure venue to house them. Coming easily has to be a function of your willingness and joy in the activity. Not that it will necessarily *be* easy, but that for you, there is a drive that is bigger and stronger than you are. For me, communicating is one of my favourite activities, assisted strongly by a love of people. I enjoy public speaking and group facilitation, and have trust in the right people being in the room with the right information flowing through me. I have largely nailed surrender in the classroom and love to observe each time I open my mouth and let the words flow out. Buddhist nun Pema Chodron recounts an anecdote about her teacher giving her instructions on how to teach. He said prepare well, know your subject, then leave your notes at the door. It's brilliant advice on how to best teach from the heart, acutely engaged with what your students want to learn, rather than what you want to teach them. So I prepare, then I surrender, and go with whatever questions and direction the students throw my way.

3. Does It Give Benefits to Others?

In the teachings of Buddhism, all of us have within us Buddha nature, and the capacity for enlightenment extends to all sentient beings. This is where mindful action and compassion are such fundaments to the teachings of living and working in your dharma. You have to have an acute awareness of your duty of care to all. In asking whether what you do fulfils that duty, there are many different ways to cut this question, so let's dig into the idea of service. Selfless service is giving freely to others.

This is the absolute bedrock that differentiates a good hustle from any old venture that has profit and personal reward as its main goal. How are *you* going to serve humanity, how is your *idea* going to serve humanity? How are you going to embed these values into your business so they stay front and centre throughout its scale and growth? This is the heart of this book—building understanding of the personal journey, preparing your mind, then preparing your capacity to execute your good hustle. Not just getting a business started, but keeping it values-based and sustainable for the term of its operation.

This is an easy one for me to apply to my venture of delivering *The Good Hustle* to the world. Within all of my products and ideas is a fail-safe route to philanthropy. I know that my skills and dharma are based on communicating and facilitating ideas that create social value. This fundamentally informs all the work I do and can conveniently be linked to earning money and raising revenue. But my endgame isn't more money and the acquisition of more stuff. Earnings translate to the funding of worthwhile projects that promote more good hustles being started. The other precious commodity is time to put towards the priceless jewel of stillness and space to pursue my spiritual practice. In my business model, once my basic costs are met (and I keep in check that they don't balloon from costs to needs to wants in a subtle First World problem escalation), all surplus funding is routed into funding social enterprises and philanthropic projects.

This model gives me a huge incentive to work harder, to serve more, to do more, driven by the knowledge of the service I can bring to other sentient beings. And as you will discover, or may have already discovered, your capacity to sell, sell, sell is boosted enormously when you completely and wholeheartedly believe in what you are doing for someone else. Knowing that every dollar is going to change a life, amplify an opportunity, or inject love and compassion into a situation, is an epic motivator.

4. Can You See Yourself Doing It For a Long Time?

Don't be confused by this, in an era of job hopping and short attention spans. Gather your answers from the previous three questions and extract the overall theme and feeling. In my case, it is sharing knowledge and hopefully wisdom—whether it is with *The Good Hustle*, or teaching yoga or supporting global start-ups; whatever the content, it is the act of a loving transmission of information that positively enables another. I can definitely say that if I was going to teach the same thing forever I would be nowhere near as sanguine about this as my path, but I can happily meander around from experience to experience transmitting the love like a satellite while my teaching channels remain diverse and interesting.

As a hangover from my early days of being a chef (where there were a lot of hangovers), I often yearn to have a little food venture somewhere to be able to dish up some tasty vegan love on a plate, to give nourishment to the world and subsidise those who can't feed themselves and their families adequately. I love cooking, feeding and serving; it comes easily, it serves humanity, all clear ticks. But I know without a shadow of a doubt that I can't do it every day. The rose-coloured food-venture fantasy fades as quickly as it comes over me, as my family and friends gently remind me of what happens when I stay in the one place day after day standing at a stove. It's off the menu for me, but happily there are lots of heart-centred entrepreneurs doing good hustles and social enterprises to meet this growing segment of the market. I can teach them how to run a great business, and cheer them on from the lip-smacking sidelines without having to tie on an apron.

Turn Your Hurdles into Hustles

Take some time now to think about your big, beautiful ideas using the Good Hustle Hurdles. Just by undertaking this exercise you will automatically exclude some concepts straight off the bat. At first this may be a little hard. There could well be some strong attachment to those concepts, and the vision of yourself in that role. But your gut will ring a bell when there are irreconcilable differences between your idea and your capacity to deliver on all of the above.

The process of having a good business idea is an iterative one. Paraphrasing Richard Branson, ideas are like buses, there is always another one coming along. We can put this in a mindfulness context and say ideas are like thoughts during meditation, there's always another one to acknowledge and dismiss. The message here is don't overthink it. If you really have to strain to fit your concept into these four noble truths of your business idea, it's not your one, and undoubtedly will be perfect for someone else. So dismiss it with love and compassion, and continue to retain the parts of it that lit you up, as this process is as heavily weighted to feeling as it is to thinking and doing.

Think of it like falling in (unconditional) love, as you have to be really, really attached to your idea to get it through the gestation period, birth it out into the market and watch it grow and take shape on its own. How do you know when you're in love? It's highly irrational, but absolutely a feeling you know when it hits you. And I don't mean the hot, lusty brain snap we have all had at one time or another that has clouded our capacity to make a good decision that can go the distance. I mean the love that you can imagine waking up with in decades to come, that is built on rock-solid foundations of honesty, respect and friendship. One that can last the distance no matter what turbulence might hit. When that idea comes along, it's likely to bug you enough that you start taking serious notice. It will buzz in your ear, tap on your shoulder, be peering in the window of your soul in a feather boa, jousting with your logical, routine and orderly life until you are ready to give it the time of day. And when that happens, you will need to be fully prepared to not only manage your mind, but to deploy it in the right mode to take you through each of the stages to get you and your idea to market.

Doing Your Business

Finding your natural state, your dharma, and from there creating a life and creativity outlet through business that reflects who you are is the central mission of *The Good Hustle*. It's a handbook to get you to a place in your mind and body where a business can emerge; a business to enable the expression of the dharma path that has lain quietly inside you, waiting for you to wake up. But much like yoga asana, you can't start with a headstand and work your way back to mountain pose. Firing up your business idea is only going to take you to the next place on your transition from caterpillar to butterfly if you are ready to fight the imaginal cells that have served you for so long, and let the part of you that has been the caterpillar die gracefully. So, wherever it is you find yourself right now, you got this. If getting up on cold mornings to meditate and do yoga, or giving up your love of cocktails to work on your business plan, or finally saying goodbye to that person or job in your life that does not serve you makes you feel sick to the stomach and emphatically say '*No*, I won't', then no means no. Don't judge yourself, or others who make different choices; you are where you are meant to be. You'll find no spiritual bullying here. Everything begins on the tip of 'I will' not 'I bloody won't and you can't make me'. But let's assume that you are at least good hustle curious. Whether or not you have been swept up in a striving frenzy of can do, or are choosing to sit this one out, it's time to have a look at some of the business tips, tricks and hacks to consider when getting your good hustle in shape. I'll cover some of the ways to merge your practice of spirituality with your business behaviour. Keeping mindfulness and motivation top of mind is essential as you go along, as this is how you are going to maintain your intention of action with meaning. And in the chapters that follow, we will discuss how to do this. By interrogating each part of your business process with the question 'Will this serve all sentient beings?', you will find you are given crystal-clear boundaries and go/no go points.

Keeping that in mind, the development of your good hustle begins with a process of ideation. This will be covered in detail in the section on the eight limbs yoga. Get your idea in clear view, and get set on it. You may be struck with a creative thunderbolt, through the previous processes I've outlined, that guides you directly to your dharma at a moment when you are ready to act. Or you may instigate the process by starting to look for the clues that lead you to your dharma: unearthing them and you on your journey of self-discovery until you end up in the same place. Whichever way, there is no better choice or better path. Only your choice and your path, only what's happening in your mind, your dharma, your attachment and your reaction. Either way, once you are there, and you have a good enough idea of what you are going to deliver through your good hustle, you will need a rough go-to-market plan.

PART THREE

THE GOOD HUSTLE PLAYBOOK

*You have to have the vision first,
the thought, then you do it.
It's so easy to stay stuck in our own little ways,
we're so scared to do something new,
we're scared to think differently.
We're scared of what the world thinks ...
be brave, do things well, think differently.*

VEN. ROBINA COURTIN, BUDDHIST NUN,
FOUNDER OF THE LIBERATION PRISON PROJECT

IN THE WEST, WE USUALLY REACH
FOR NEW KNOWLEDGE, BURYING OURSELVES
DEEPER IN INFORMATION,
WITHOUT REALISING THAT WE ARE ALREADY
FULL OF THOUGHTS AND WORDS AND
OPINIONS, BUT LIGHT ON WISDOM.

The Good Hustle Toolbox

The who's, why's, what's and how's have been defined and revealed. You've spent some time on a first date with your mind and haven't snuck out a bathroom window to get away. You've stuck up some posters on telegraph poles to help find your missing Buddha nature and a great business idea. You're loaded on growth mindset and with effort and resilience nothing is out of your reach. It's time to get practical. Yes, more practical than you've ever imagined. And to do that, it's time to integrate our new practices with a framework to deliver you a working model of your next big thing.

Lean In to a Lean Start

The lean start-up process is a continuous cycle based on three repeating phases: build, measure and learn. Good business planning is a continuous cycle based on three similar repeating phases: plan, review and revise. The two work together collaboratively to produce a blueprint for managing the nimble business of now, both digital and bricks and mortar. This is for many the single hardest part of the start-up process. If you haven't had much to do with the world of business, and are feeling clueless about where to begin, this can be where you yield to the temptation to abandon ship, and make a whole tonne of excuses why letting the moment go through to the keeper is a better idea than tackling a business plan. Of course it's not. And remember, wisdom is learning through doing. No one was born with a silver business plan in their mouth, and at some point everyone has to work one out. We're not inventing anything new, and the good news is that it's much easier than you might think. We've already talked about the value of the lean business model, and of course there is also a lean business plan to go with it. The one I use the most to demonstrate the simplicity of what you really need to know is Chris Guillebeau's *$100 Startup* business plan one-pager.

Extracted from Chris' excellent book *The $100 Startup* (which is a dharma manifesto if ever there was one), the business plan proves that less is more. You can grab a copy of it gratis at 100startup.com and it basically asks you, in one page, no more, to answer the following questions in one or two sentences: 'What will you sell? Who will buy it? How will your business idea help people? What will you charge? How will you get paid? How will customers learn about your business? How can you encourage referrals?' Once these foundations are established, some measurements of benchmark success are posed including whether the success metrics will measure the number of customers, or focus on the annual net income, or something else. Then it asks you to do a little troubleshooting and risk management. Time to get those deep-seated fears out onto the page and look for an answer—if one exists, which at this time in the planning cycle it may not.

Next, you need to note down any worries or questions, and how you plan to solve or answer them. Choose your three most burning issues and address them; just the act of doing this will make you feel better about the things you don't know. And with your new training of surrender and faith in the timing and the dharma, you can leave the answers to be revealed in their own sweet time. Know that risk is there, and will always be there; some risk will be able to be controlled, some not. Rather than trying to eliminate it, accept that there is never 100 per cent certainty in anything (except death). Make sure you are comfortable with all of the potential outcomes of the risks you can think of. The other thing you can be pretty sure about is that whatever situations arise, they will be impermanent and somehow you will manage them. Everyone's appetite for risk will be different. The belief in the risk likelihood will be different. Once you have had a shot at what you think the big issues are likely to be, you can bring in your close circle of collaborators and pressure test your thinking with a wider group.

The next question in Chris' one-page business plan is a good one: 'How else will you make money from this project?' I like the way he phrases this with 'how else', as he is shining a light on the opportunities that flow from action. So growth mindset. What could develop in the future? What scope is there for other products or services to emerge from this original concept? This leads to broader thinking, such as whether you could charge to train other people in your method. Are there franchise or wholesale opportunities? Is there an innovative method or packaging you've created that has commercial value or intellectual property (IP) in its own right? This is the nudge to continue the creative process you began when refining your idea at the start. But remember, crawling, walking and running—in that order. With some stop-offs for meditation, yoga and meaningful conversations with future customers of course!

Your Mission and Vision (Should You Choose to Accept It)

While I like Guillebeau's method and use it all the time to help my clients get their structure down, there are two other things in our good hustle framework that are essential at the beginning of our business plan. These are the vision and mission statements. You want to have these in your planning documents as they clearly articulate the motivation for the business. They may be seen by some as a 'fluffy' addition to your documents; however, in the case of a good hustle, the reason why we are doing what we are doing is the motivation: it is the central nervous system of the business case. There are differences between vision and mission and how you write them up. The mission is why you exist. It is one succinct, dynamic statement, about a sentence long, detailing why you exist. The best mission statements are clear, compelling and concise. Longer than fifteen words and you are getting into essay territory. Nailing the mission statement is tricky in the sense that any perfect one-liner takes time to get right. Each word has to be powerful and economical, so give yourself time and space to be 100 per cent happy with what you create. Sit with it, meditate on it, pick it apart and put it back together. The good news is that once done, this also serves as your elevator pitch and networking intro—you'll soon know it like the back of your hand and be able to reel it off with conviction.

Best practice is always that the message of what, for who and why is absolutely unambiguous. The reason this is such a good double down for your elevator pitch is that when you get the opportunity to spread the word of what you are doing, especially with someone who may have the capacity to help you grow, you need to get their attention and keep it. If it looks like you are wobbling and are unsure of the business case yourself, then you won't inspire confidence in your capacity to deliver.

Vision can be simply defined as what your company aspires to be; which can be quite different from what your company is, as represented by your mission statement. When done right, your vision statement should help drive decisions and goals in your company. By doing the work crafting words that represent and reflect the dharma of the good hustle you are creating, you are weaving a brand narrative for you and your customers, and really beginning to make the idea move from being inside your head to something tangible.

It's not essential, but while you are on a roll with your underpinning statements, this could be a good time to pen some core values. Core values are what support the vision, shape the culture, and reflect you and your business values. They are your principles, beliefs or philosophy. Make yourself a list of about five things, and bind them to your mission and vision.

Evolving Your Business Plan

Using lean start-up principals doesn't mean skipping the business planning, or jumping in without direction or guidance. It means starting small with a business plan that summarises the current strategy, metrics, milestones, tasks and basic responsibilities. It's not the doorstop-sized output of an MBA or a printed and bound document you show to your bank manager then never use again.

A real business plan should be agile and grow organically, just like a lean start-up. The process starts with a concrete and specific plan for what's supposed to happen, and continues forever. It needs regular review and revision as the market, customers and, in the case of good hustle, your increasing clarity on the direction of your dharma inform it.

One of the great benefits of using the lean start-up model as an entrepreneur is that, as you are working on your mind management practice, it roots out the paralysis of perfectionism. If you are stuck in being the doer, never being enough, and worrying continually about reputational damage or being criticised, the likelihood of you taking the leap to actually opening your doors, digital or tangible, is limited. Having an agile business plan and limitless opportunity to be able to improve and change salves the idea that things can always be better, while allowing the action of being a good hustle to begin.

I've talked up *The $100 Startup* one-page business plan, but don't take my word for it. Maybe you want something that is more detailed. Give Google a whirl and find the best template for you to step out the beginnings of your good hustle. Avoid anything that wants five-year projections, as this doesn't suit the lean framework (or reality). Just plan the time it takes to get to the market launch, and about six months out from that, maximum. Don't forget your budgets and detailed cost breakdowns. These are important to ascertain whether what you want to do is financially doable and, more critically, sustainable. Then keep that rolling as you grow and develop.

Share this complete document with your trusted group of fans, ask for feedback, collaborate and be open, embracing the guidance. With your idea firmly in your back pocket, and a business plan mapped out, now you need to think about what your MVP will involve.

Minimum Viable Products

A minimum viable product (or MVP) for your good hustle is the product or service with just those features (and not more) that allow you to ship (or sell through bricks and mortar, or digitally deliver) a product that your first customers or early adopters can see and use, will pay money for, and, most importantly, give you feedback on. Again, no need to put your panic pants on. If you are going into a spin thinking you aren't even finished reading the book and now you've got to create an MVP, this is just a heads-up that you don't have to wait and sequentially develop everything. As you are planning and meditating and preparing yourself for your dharma-driven launch, be thinking about getting out there and into the market, and envision what that tangibly looks like.

When I was writing my book *Dogs of India*, I wanted to seed the idea of the book into the minds of people so that when it was done, they were already excited and wanted more. I built a website and started talking about the story, the characters, the writer's journey, and the book's philanthropic mission of funding vet care for stray Indian dogs. When I had some writing that I was happy with, I released sample chapters. This was effectively an MVP—it was just those features that allow potential clients to get interested, leading to the ultimate goal of a book purchase down the track. You can see your MVP as the next level in your commitment to living your dharma, where, as they say, shit gets real. Trust in your gift and your belief, and the work you are doing. Let the MVP be a gulp of clean, oxygen-rich air after being down the mines your whole life.

Putting together a website or, even leaner, a landing page, is one way of getting an MVP out there. You have plenty of choice in whether you make your own using a template cloud-based service, get a freelancer to design one or use a full-service agency. These are all decisions you can make based on budget, need and the functionality requirements of your business. Just know that you will need something, and it will be the link for all of your social media channels, and the place where all your online transactions can happen quickly and easily for your customers. You could choose to do as I did and have a website that was at first just a homepage with info about me and the book, and a blog. The blog will give you a hook to get people coming back and becoming familiar with you, your brand and your values, where you can start building the conversation.

If your business idea is in the tangible realm—say, you were wanting to run yoga classes—these too can have MVPs (and of course need a digital presence to get your people following along). Find a studio that will give you a slot on their timetable, or a suitable empty space or sunny park to launch your yoga class to the world. Describe it and your unique selling point (USP) via your digital channels, then promote, execute and gather feedback from participants. There you have an MVP for a yoga class. For food businesses—say you want to have your own vegan street-food truck or cafe—you don't have to wait until you can purchase your food truck or get a lease. Find a commercial kitchen that can rent you some time—look for schools or clubs with certified kitchens; many of them will happily let you use theirs for reasonable prices. Create your products, and take them to the people via markets, pop-ups, take-overs of other people's cafes, or even host your own party at home where people come to sample your treats and give feedback. An MVP doesn't have to be complex, it is just a method of taking early samples of what you do, to who you do it for.

Be It Till You Are It

'Fake it till you make it' is an expression I detest. It's problematic to me because of the word 'fake'. When starting a new business, you are learning new information, mastering new skills with the discipline of practice—totally growth mindset territory. This is about as real an experience as you can get, with no faking involved. No doubt you are already feeling like you are about to be called out at any minute by real professionals on your ignorance and lack, which drives fear and shame. Faking it till you make it is fundamentally all about what other people think of you; it is trying to keep a front of reputation for a faceless crowd, so you can backfill it and eventually be that big gal on campus. Using an MVP allows you to take people on the journey with you from day one and let them experience it—in its full reality of challenge and triumph. Falling flat on your face is an act of leadership, as it encourages all of the people who are too trapped to do what you are doing to believe in themselves and their capacity. As you are an agile, nimble business, your end product will probably be some distance from these early iterations anyway; and it is great to be able to reflect on where you started, and reward those early adopters that have been on the journey from the start. All of which will provide you with a history of your efforts, and the tale of your dharma in development. MVPs are in this way an excellent reminder of impermanence. Good hustlers don't fake it till they make it. I like to have a different spin on it: be it till you are it. That way you are always it, just in a perpetual process of becoming.

Your Digital Strategy

MVP sorted, sitting alongside it is your lean but live business plan. The final element of this triple gem of good hustle planning tools is your digital strategy, which will enable the engagement of your idea/MVP with the market. You've already got the what and why in your business plan and MVP, now it's time for the how. Managing your digital strategy when you are developing your good hustle starts with having a strategy. Like the name says, a digital strategy is a document where you consider all of the elements of your digital and online suite of marketing tools, and how you are going to apply them to building your business. When building a digital marketing strategy, it's important to think upfront about what you are trying to achieve. Is it designed to increase brand awareness? Is it to drive sales? Is it to educate your market to remove barriers to the previous two, or is it perhaps all three? To do this, you need to truly understand what your customer wants, what makes your offering unique and the most direct way to connect with your customers.

Writing a digital strategy for your business is not as intimidating as it sounds. It's just a document outlining how your business should handle the different aspects of digital, from the website and mobile to email, social media and digital marketing. Like the epic five-year business plan, creating a digital strategy that looks three to five years ahead is unrealistic—technology just moves too fast. Equally, accurate budgeting is difficult when the landscape is evolving at such a rapid rate. A digital strategy, like your lean business plan, takes a different approach. It doesn't need to cover everything in great depth, but instead should cover a time span of six to twelve months of implementable actions linked to a calendar of events, with clear measurements and points of decision. A digital strategy needs to focus more on creating a detailed roadmap to enable the right decisions on your marketing campaign spend, rather than defining everything up front. The exact scope of your digital strategy will vary depending on your business and what you do.

You do need to write the strategy with a budget in mind. With a clear budget established you will know what the priorities are, and which recommendations will need to be implemented incrementally. As the digital environment is constantly evolving, this is a sensible, agile approach to how you develop, implement, measure and evolve your tools to suit your business and customer needs. This acknowledges that, like your product and service development, your digital assets are never finished, and digital expenditure is ongoing rather than a one-off spend.

The digital strategy for your business is part of your business strategy, and in many cases when the business is wholly online, the digital strategy *is* your business strategy. Assuming you have read the previous section and have a lean business plan that isn't a dusty doorstop, the digital strategy can sit within the marketing, sales and communication section, much like the Bhagavad Gita is a smaller but critical part of the *Mahabharata*, and can stand alone or be read as part of the whole. Your digital strategy relies heavily on a very clear understanding of your customers, competitors and the value proposition of your good hustle. The information that is created by knowing these three elements guides your strategy to target the digital channels where your customers/clients are likely to hang out. Are they badass galpreneurs on Facebook and Instagram? Professionals on LinkedIn? Fast-moving tech junkies on Twitter? Global opinion leaders on WeChat, Hipsters on Snapchat or maybe designers and bloggers on Pinterest? Do they want video, mobile, shareable gifs and memes, chock-a-block shops with seamless pay gateways, deep-diving blogs or pretty infographics—or perhaps a combination of all of these things? To know how to talk to your people, you have to know them, and really get what motivates their lives. Let the sense of your ideal customer percolate in your mind. This is how you will know and refine the needs of your customers and be able to focus on delivering communications and interactions that best suit their way of engaging.

The Value Proposition

In regards to the business side of *The Good Hustle* we need to talk about money. Or more specifically, the value proposition. 'How much do I charge?' is a big question for new entrepreneurs, but the real question they are asking is 'What am I worth?' Developing a price strategy is an important part of working out how and if you can make money from your brilliant idea. This is kinda critical. The best ideas are only good insofar as they are able to cost recover sufficiently to keep staff employed, doors open, the power on, and make you a living wage. That you may end up not being able to make enough money to green light your idea doesn't mean it isn't good, or that there isn't a needy user base crying out for it. All too often it is a great idea that will meet a gap, but the business model isn't apparent and there is no capacity to make money by doing it. Timing can play into this, as whatever factor is making it unviable could change, opening up an opportunity. If you have been working through your idea while you've been reading, and are getting a sinking feeling that there are a few insurmountable risks, this may well be a good time for some assessment of viability.

To understand the value proposition more deeply, let's start with a basic product-based business. You have to take into account the cost of base inputs (including your time), as well as packaging, marketing and transport. Don't forget postage if you aren't selling direct. Costs of things like market stalls and their collateral have to be included here too, and your time standing on that stall, as that eight hours plus travel time isn't free. If you are entering a world where you need a workshop or a manufacturing centre or retail space, you obviously have to factor everything at this scale. When you can work out the unit cost, then you need to work out what the market will pay. Look around for similar examples at the high and low end of the market and get a feel for where yours fits.

You've established what it costs to produce, and what the market will pay for it. The difference is your profit. Now multiply that by the volume you expect to sell weekly, monthly, annually. Is it enough to keep you living happily? It is a simple equation, and the important part is that you be really strict about all the input costs, and look honestly at the viability. Once your base is established, you can work out if there are things like upsells, premium deals, or discounts for multiples that will create different pricing tiers. Don't be afraid to ask people who are already in your sector about their business models and costs. Many entrepreneurs will be more than happy to give you a hand and help you avoid rookie pitfalls.

If you are selling a service, then you need to work out how you are going to charge: by the hour, by the job, on a retainer, on a subscription or using a tiered approach. Again, what should direct this thinking is the research you do first to see what your customers want. How do they prefer to pay? Ask people what they think the service you are proposing is worth; would they like less or more, and if so, of what? There is no better source than the very people who are going to be your purchasers, so ask and then listen to what they say. This is a critical part of the MVP process, too. Do your research on what is being offered in your industry, what the common price points are, and where you might fit. I always caution against low pricing because of a perceived 'newness' to the industry. That is your insecurity rather than what the market thinks you are worth. It is always harder to raise prices once you have begun, so do your homework, and land on a price that gives you enough, makes your customers feel as though they are getting great value and, most importantly, covers your costs sustainably into the future. The bottom line is to give more value than the customer perceives they are paying for. This fits perfectly in a good hustle model, as you are made to give service and value, willingly and with love. If your baseline is covered, then simply work out what will be the cherry on the top of the love sundae with regard to how much profit you need to comfortably survive and give back.

As flagged, some of you may be in situations where your idea looks as though it is going to be unfeasible. If you are convinced that the idea needs pursuing, really start to interrogate sources of revenue, input costs and who will pay for the product, from as many angles as possible. This type of dilemma is especially apparent for good hustles that are serving a needy user group where the customer is not paying for the service. The temptation is often to start up by getting a grant, with the assumption that other funding will be forthcoming. While this approach is within the spirit of good hustling—to surrender and have faith—the better path of valour is to establish a business that has a clear pathway to sustainable revenue, so vulnerable users are not left high and dry when the funding runs out. I'm talking here about organisations with overheads and fixed costs, that can't be run in a nimble and agile way. If the original business model isn't working when you do the sums, how can you find another way to deliver the outcomes? Can you simplify the business? Can you offer a narrower service and reduce the fixed costs? Don't rush in, allow yourself to think through all the options as far outside the box as you can go.

Allow the spaciousness to find a solution. It could be that you desperately want to help women who are victims of domestic violence. A shelter is your dream, but the costs of getting a space, and staffing, insurance and the like are well beyond your capacity. You believe it's your dharma and your calling, so what are your options? The first steps may simply be to volunteer your services at a shelter, and see if you can satisfy your need to help this way, plus it will help you hone your ideas about what is needed, from the frontline. Maybe look at what women undergoing homelessness and/or domestic abuse need in a practical sense, and provide things like food, clothes, laundry services, hairdressing, childcare, movie tickets or personal products. What services could you offer? Shelter is obviously a big part of what women in this situation require, but there are many other ways of offering valuable support that require far less upfront investment. This is just one example of how to work around the problem of not having a long-term, sustainable solution to your good hustle. There is always another way; the question comes back to the core of what you are trying to achieve. Follow your curiosity and trust in the answer showing up. The question is 'How can I best serve?'

I strongly caution against starting up your idea and waiting for a funding miracle. From my own painful experience on a number of boards that have faced this exact dilemma, I know this doesn't always end well. Good hustles are not immune to failure because they are heart centred. These types of ventures are probably more vulnerable because the drive is not purely fiscal, and sometimes the more traditional business planning underpinnings are ignored at the outset; these are things that are virtually impossible to reverse-engineer.

Knowing and recognising your value, and making sure that your needs are met, is a baseline in sustainability. You may find that you can survive on much less income than you were used to. It is common to hear people talk about how much smaller their lives could become, how much simpler and happier, once they let go of all of the grasping and attachments. In *The $100 Startup*, Chris Guillebeau suggests that in your first year of trading you should make the equivalent of the minimum wage in your country your baseline.

While a good hustle comes from a place of creating value for others through unconditional love and service, it is mandatory that you are able to earn enough revenue to make it a viable business. You know what you need as your starting point to be able to launch. I encourage you to get as creative as possible in finding ways to begin as frugally as possible. The aim is to transition into a place where you are living in your dharma while delivering service to humanity, in whatever small or large way you conceive that gift. It is always easier to innovate, scale and grow once you are rolling. This is why the MVP is such a great approach to get you in the game. Starving in the process is not a viable option.

Your value is always the combination of your needs being met by the surplus from the costs of what you are selling, and the price the market is willing to pay. When possible, keep your fixed costs low at the outset, and prove your idea in the nimblest and most agile way before you commit to anything that is going to drive your costs up. Keep taking action, keep talking to your customers, keep looking for ways to do what you do better, to deliver more value and bring in more revenue so you have more to share around. The key ideas here are sustainability—for you and your customers—and being of service, however you are able to best deliver that with what you've got.

Delivering Happiness

Zappos CEO Tony Hseih literally and metaphorically wrote the book on customer service. It's called *Delivering Happiness*, and it chronicles his experience as a successful entrepreneur of dotcom booms one and two, making billions of dollars along the way. Tony Hseih had the revelation after his first multi-million dollar exit from LinkExchange, an online advertising business he co-founded, that money didn't buy him anything but more stuff. His pursuit became creating the ultimate work environment that gave people the freedom to be themselves, and in doing so the freedom to turn their attention 100 per cent to customer service. Hsieh knows that when people are serving others, they are happy, and the by-product is incredibly high rates of return customers and evangelistic word of mouth.

When retailers complain about online taking their sales, I always argue that no one ever chooses to wait for a product on price alone, when they can have instant gratification through fantastic customer service and perhaps pay a little more. They will, however, forgo the gratification if they perceive that the service is poor and the cost is higher. Zappos' model of online delivery doesn't promise that they are the cheapest, they just promise exceptional customer service. The product is secondary in importance to the experience of truly being served as far as that corporate culture is concerned.

Good hustles are defined by a number of elements, but the principal one is that the hustle is undertaken in service to others. The companion to customer service is a commitment to ensuring that service is embedded in every part of the business, and is the backbone of the culture you are creating. You can't successfully run a good hustle unless everyone who is part of that business is in it for the same reasons. Earlier in this chapter we looked at mission and value statements. These documents have to be the answer to every question your business poses in the set-up and operational stage. Will this decision, hire or investment deliver the mission and values of this business? In the next section of this book we are going to turn to Patanjali's Yoga Sutras, and set out how the ancient sages systematically approached the path to enlightenment, using the eight limbs as a way of framing their actions against a values compass. Your actions as an individual will determine the culture of your company, far more strongly than any set of values you stick up on the wall. In *Delivering Happiness*, Tony Hseih says, 'Just figure out what your personal values are then just make those the corporate values.' The key here is that you have to figure them out. You may think you know what your values are, but until you test them in the kinds of fast-moving situations you will face when getting your good hustle running, you won't really know for sure. Work out who your customer is, who you are serving, and then build your business model around how best to deliver happiness to them. Walk in their shoes as best as you can, understand the minutiae of their fears and hopes and how what you do in your good hustle can make some element of their lives easier and better. Remember, you don't have to change the world, you just have to make it better for someone else for a moment, then repeat that action endlessly.

Managing Your Mind

You've got the tools and the template to sort your ideas. Keep working on them, giving them time and space to incubate. While they are bubbling away, let's continue to understand tools for the management of the mind, which, as outlined, is such a critical canon in the management of business. Yet, despite having written curricula and taught in undergraduate and MBA university courses, I've never seen it even casually mentioned in relation to business mastery. For aspiring entrepreneurs, the mind is the beginning and the end of the story; when the mind is a collaborative partner on the business journey, the path to achieving anything is infinitely easier. To wrestle the mind into the right shape for contentment, we are going to take a look at some ancient wisdoms and apply them to our contemporary situations. One of those concerns an epic battle, both of place and of the mind: the battle of Kurukshetra. This battle is the backdrop for the epic Sanskrit tale the *Mahabharata*, that, as mentioned, the classic book of yoga, the Bhagavad Gita, is lifted from. The Gita is essentially a series of *slokas* or verses that document a conversation between Prince Arjuna and Lord Krishna—Arjuna's charioteer, friend and wise council (and, conveniently for Arjuna, a god in human form).

Where once executives read *The Art of War* to learn leadership, the times and behaviours are a changing. The Gita is a text relevant for today as a frank discussion about how to push through doubt and uncertainty and fulfil dharma. Similarly, the Yoga Sutras, despite both the texts being authored centuries ago, speak to the transcendent nature of our problems and anxieties with clear remedies for how to fix what ails us. I said at the outset of this book that if we really wanted to shift from our lives of attachment and suffering, the recipe was already available with a number of variations leading to the same path. These two texts, both essential in the Vedic canon and in the lives of billions of Indians and Westerners, take different approaches to the same destination.

Buddha, or Siddhartha Gautama as he was back then, was revealing his enlightened teachings some 700 years before Patanjali's Yoga Sutras, the individual teachings of which are said to have numbered in excess of 84,000. He too saw people engaged in struggle, experiencing suffering and stress, and looked for a way to relieve them. The Gita, the Yoga Sutras and Buddha's teachings all have a single central nervous system: when the mind is managed through various practices, suffering is diminished. The end point of it all for Krishna, Patanjali and Buddha is for us to attain liberation or illumination of the mind, which leads to choices that create peace and equanimity for ourselves, and for others.

The management of the mind needs wisdom as its fuel. In the West, we usually reach for new knowledge, burying ourselves deeper in information, without realising that we are already full of thoughts and words and opinions, but light on wisdom. Thinking tends to enmesh us in more thoughts, deepening the mire of confusion rather than lessening it. Wisdom is not a result of thoughts and philosophy; rather, it comes as insight gained from direct experience about how life works, applied to our own lives.

The Bhagavad Gita prescribes a way through yogic practice to be free from mental anguish and suffering. It serves as both an ancient and compelling story of Krishna leading Arjuna into battle, and a spiritual text on the inner struggle for self-mastery and the attainment of happiness through yoga. The story of the Gita begins on a battlefield, at the cusp of a colossal war between two large families, the Kauravas and Arjuna's family, the Pandavas. The families are mired in the hatred and mistrust that the grasping of inheritance and assets can bring. Arjuna is distraught as he looks across the battle lines. He knows that by engaging in this war, hundreds of family members and friends will be lost on both sides of the fight. Arjuna is faced with a personal and ethical crisis, which he is unwilling and unable to solve. Krishna is a childhood friend of Arjuna's and, with his spiritual powers as an incarnation of the Hindu Lord Vishnu, he has a broader view of the need for Arjuna to experience the suffering of battle to discover his true nature of self. The resulting conversation between Arjuna and Krishna is used as a discourse on the purpose of one's life, and the path of yoga as a tool to unravel the type of paralysing anguish that Arjuna is experiencing. Krishna is conveying a solution both allegorical and practical for Arjuna and all readers who are similarly faced with paralysing and seemingly intractable problems.

The sage Patanjali also promoted mastery of the mind as an essential practice towards pure awareness of the perfection of our own divinity. What Patanjali was prescribing was not more learning, or more religion, he simply presented a training program of practice to release us from the pains of being human. Buddha had his own training program, which looked remarkably like Patanjali's—clean and empty the mind with meditation, release yourself from false perceptions, still down, and witness your own perfection and innate wisdom as a path to assist all others to reach enlightenment. Krishna recommended meditation and action, which I have adopted for the yoga of business. Such meditation, Krishna admits in the Gita, is difficult, but, growth mindset style, one can achieve it through sustained effort. The yogi must learn to meditate continually, and make their mind one-pointed, restricting any extraneous thoughts or sensual distractions. The yogi should practise such meditation for their own purification only—without any ulterior motive. This contemplative form of yoga, systematised in Patanjali's eight limbs, is the form of yoga that is ultimately going to control the mind.

The point of giving all of this background to the Yoga Sutras, Gita and the teachings of the Buddha is to underscore that the afflictions that trouble us today are not new. They are not even a little bit retro. They are positively ancient and have been exhibited by humans across continents throughout recorded history. I see this as a relieving and motivating fact. In the quest to lose the 'I' of the ego and merge into greater loving consciousness with all my fellow humans, it is good to know that we, in this current generation, are not alone in feeling the way we do. We have not caused the downfall of happiness with the interwebs or lost the capacity for loving awareness over the last century, although we have given it a pretty good shot. We are simply in the present, in the thick of it and, because of our limited perceptions and raging egos, are taking full ownership of it, reactively and painfully. Each epoch no doubt had their own version of where we are now, and at the precipice of their despair it would have felt like the darkest hour.

What Happens in Samvega ...

Buddhists have a word to describe the place of seeking that I suspect will be an a-ha moment of relief in your self-diagnosis. It certainly was for me when I came across it in author and yogi Stephen Cope's excellent book *The Wisdom of Yoga*. That word is 'samvega'. Cope, quoting

Buddhist monk Thanissaro Bhikkhu, describes samvega as three clusters of feelings occurring simultaneously: shock, alienation and dismay at the futility and meaninglessness of life. This manifests as a sense of our own culpability, complacency and, to a degree, foolishness in being so blind to this situation; and a sense of anxiety coupled with urgency to get out of this messy, meaningless cycle and evolve to a new level of meaning and awareness.

Sound familiar?

I'm surprised that samvega doesn't get more of a run in the adoption of Buddhism in the West. We can't turn round without hearing the word mindfulness (which of course is a great thing for mainstreaming meditation), but having the language to describe the cluster of despair, futility and urgency for change that samvega brings us would be a salve when the road gets rough for many of us. Samvega is linked to the moment where we see material aspirations to be empty in their capacity to deliver lasting happiness or true satisfaction. This is usually a radical realisation, and one that deconstructs everything that we have been raised on and worked towards; the messages of our culture and marketing experts; and the narratives about ourselves we have bought into. It is an unravelling that is swift, deep and awkward. Samvega is uncomfortable, and is probably akin to what we would describe as a midlife crisis. It is aptly a product of mid life, as in early life we are striving to get to the fun bit where all the work and suffering pay off. By mid life, we suddenly realise there is no one coming to save us. The usual demonstration of this trio of dismay is a desperate acquisition of new items of desire such as sports cars, new breasts or younger partners, followed by a penchant for numbing substances.

I hazard there is a less visible cohort of people who, when they hit this period, don't consume to relieve the pain but are driven to turn within, and to look for guidance on how to access their true nature of self. We want to become quiet, away from all the noise that has masked the early squeaks and clanks of the wheels beginning to fall off. Where midlife crisis in the Western context implies breakdown, shame and public humiliation and a gradual acceptance of the inevitability of death and aging, samvega in contrast is a necessary and welcome step to awareness. We can't go from zero to awake at the speed of light. All of the processes outlined in the Gita, the noble truths and the eight limbs of the Yoga Sutras are undertaken as a practice over time, once the awareness of the false perceptions of objects as happiness has occurred. Rather than being a state of emergency, it is a stage of emergence. It is at this point of meeting samvega that many of us start to seriously look at what we are doing with our lives and wondering whether we could do more that is meaningful and feeds our souls. The answer of course is yes; the answer is starting a good hustle, and your questioning why and how is the underpinning motivation of this book.

Samvega appears in Buddhist teachings, and was also referenced by Patanjali in the first chapter of the Sutras—he could obviously see that this emergence of awareness was the catalyst for change. He characterises it as a vehement determination to find our way out of suffering. This vehemence is required to muster the necessary passion to catapult oneself out of the road of crisis and stasis into action and change, even if that action is initially undertaken in a quiet and still form, like meditation. I vividly remember reading the chapter in Stephen Cope's book where I first met samvega. I was in India, in Rishikesh, at a very damp, mouldy ashram overlooking the Ganges. After a couple of torrid days of 'welcome to India' gastro, I wobbled outside and forded the stream of sadhus with their hands out for alms. Desperate to eat a piece of solid food, I saw in front of me, like a mirage, a German bakery. Next to the bakery was a bookstore with plenty of bootleg English language titles and *The Wisdom of Yoga* grabbed my attention in my weakened state of seeking.

As I read the description of samvega, it completely reflected the feeling I'd had for a couple of frustrating years before I left my formal executive roles: a combination of deep, anger-fuelled frustration, of anguish about the futility and is-this-all-there-is-ness about my life, and the increasingly hysterical cries from my heart to be shown that this wasn't what my precious life was going to deliver to the world. I felt trapped, and in me was the growing kernel of determination to find my way out of the pointlessness of my suffering. My difficulty was that I was trying to think my way out of a problem that lived in my mind. I was the embodiment of knowledge without wisdom. It seems pretty funny now. I suspect many of us do enlightenment like this, as we huff and puff through endless sun salutations and strive for yogic prowess while our minds whir like crazy, creating more problems to solve.

The expression 'First World problems' is really our self-deprecating way of acknowledging that we are culturally experiencing samvega. Our wealth, craving, attachment and meaningless existence flash up on the billboard of our day-to-day lives and we don't like what we see. So we trivialise it with a throwaway line and return to being the life of a party that we aren't sure we wanted to stay at quite so long. The problem with the Western experience of samvega is the amplification of ridiculousness when you are in a mire of misery, surrounded by wealth. It is hard to whine 'There must be more than this', when there is ample coverage of all basic and not-so-basic needs. We are buried underneath our things, often piling more fuel, of possessions and material goods, onto a fire that is already a raging inferno. What would extinguish the fire? Only the cooling stillness of turning in, shutting the eyes, removing the stimulus, and beginning the long, slow process of decoupling from those false perceptions.

PART FOUR

THE YOGA OF BUSINESS

It is better to fail at your own dharma than succeed at the dharma of someone else.

KRISHNA, BHAGAVAD GITA

ESPECIALLY WHEN ON THAT NERVOUS, EXCITED CUSP OF STARTING SOMETHING NEW, THE TEMPTATION IS TO WALLOW IN ENDLESS LEARNING. WOMEN ARE REPEAT OFFENDERS IN BELIEVING THAT THEY NEED MORE AND MORE KNOWLEDGE TO BE ABLE TO SUCCESSFULLY EXECUTE A BUSINESS IDEA. YOU HAVE TO LOOK OUT FOR THE POINT AT WHICH THE QUEST FOR KNOWLEDGE BECOMES A SAFE HAVEN FOR DOING NOTHING AND AVOIDING WISDOM. ... WHEN ALL THE BOOKS ARE READ, PODCASTS ARE LISTENED TO, BLOGS ARE SCANNED AND TWEETS AND POSTS CONSUMED, THERE IS A POINT AT WHICH YOU HAVE TO RELY ON YOUR OWN WISDOM AND BEGIN.

Now, the Teachings of Yoga ...

And so begins the opening line of Patanjali's Yoga Sutras. It's simple and profound, with an almost theatrical flourish. In this final section of *The Good Hustle* it is time to delve into the eight limbs of yoga as prescribed by Patanjali, and link them to our progress along the pathway to creating a good hustle of our own. You may feel somewhat overwhelmed right about now. Your newly diagnosed samvega is no doubt in overdrive, and as you look across your life, over the piles of people, things, responsibilities, to-dos and should'ves, you may well feel that a new business or even just an idea will be the butterfly's wing that sets off the avalanche you've been narrowly avoiding.

This is how you should feel, as you are, metaphorically, at the rubbish dump, witnessing the massive yellow excavator plough through the trash of your mind accumulated over a lifetime. You will no doubt be clinging strongly in places to your favourite bits. As I said at the outset, the heavy lifting for becoming a modern yogi in life and in business is all in the mindset. The rest flows gently from the establishment of good practices, keeping in mind the mind is everything.

The first step at the beginning of your good hustle is to investigate the difference between a good good hustle and a bad good hustle.

What ('s) a Good Idea

The process of ideation, especially when it comes to creating a meaningful life that delivers service and value to the world, is a sequential process. The idea has to be created, it has to have compelling commercial potential—even (and especially) if it is applied to a social good where the impact will be more valuable than ever. You have to be able to identify a market for the idea, and you have to be able to deliver it to that market in a way that is suitable and simple. On a personal level, you have to be able to manage risk, and have a business model that combines your idea with the skills needed to realise it. You also need to have the capacity to source or generate adequate funding to keep you and your business afloat until sufficient revenue kicks in. These steps, as I'll demonstrate in the following pages, can work in tandem with your personal journey through Patanjali's eight limbs of yoga. This work is infinitely easier when you have the structure of ethical and moral guidance that being yogi delivers, along with the capacity to surrender to your internal divinity, your ancient wisdom and your sense of what will serve others best, without diminishing your own capacity for happiness and peace.

Meet the Ashtangas

To help you to grasp and assimilate the eight limbs of yoga as outlined by Patanjali in the Yoga Sutras, I'm going to link them to the process of taking an idea from concept to market entry. But first, let us meet the ashtanga family. The 'ashta' (eight) 'anga' (limbs) of yoga basically act as guidelines on how to live a meaningful and purposeful life. Beginning with 'yama' (restraints), then followed by 'niyama' (observances), 'asana' (postures), 'pranayama' (breathing), 'pratyahara' (turning within), 'dharana' (concentration), 'dhyana' (meditation) and 'samadhi' (union with the divine), the eight limbs are laid out as though you are walking along an overgrown path and finding new clues in a treasure hunt to discover your own true nature of self. While they look linear to our Western way of thinking, you may of course backtrack, or head up an unmarked path, or camp out for a while at a spot where you feel comfortable before you set off again. You may want to light a flare and get airlifted out at moments where you feel your comfort zone being grossly infringed. But once the light is shone a little further in front of you, you will want to keep exploring, as your curiosity will light up and you will want to know what is around that next limb. The eight limbs of yoga provide an incredibly handy set of guidelines to work with, and if you use them as such, they become an invaluable framework of values and actions for your good hustle to begin, to flourish, and to benefit others.

1. The Yamas

The first limb, yama (which has five sub-limbs), deals with our ethical standards and sense of integrity, focusing on our behaviour and how we conduct ourselves. Yamas are also known as the restraints and relate to our engagement with the external world. The yamas act as a clearing and cleaning tool on the path to dharma being revealed. It's important that the contemporary context for who and how we are today in our Western condition is woven into the yamas. This softens the precepts and makes them more accessible to our daily experience. Both the yamas and niyamas (or observances) serve as a prescription for moral and ethical conduct and self-discipline and they help us to acknowledge the spiritual aspects of our nature.

There are five yamas: 'ahimsa' (nonviolence), 'satya' (truthfulness), 'asteya' (non-stealing), 'brahmacharya' (continence/chastity) and 'aparigraha' (non-covetousness or non-grasping). Don't let the unfamiliar Sanskrit words distract you from their message; in a growth mindset way it's just more fun language for you to learn and grow your brain with.

i) Ahimsa

Ahimsa is a relatively common understanding in and outside of yoga circles. Translated as nonviolence, it can be widely interpreted; from mindfulness with every step so as not to harm a tiny insect under our feet, to conscious eating with the welfare of all living creatures in mind, to the avoidance of combat with our fellow humans. When you are thinking sentient beings and your duty of care, this is ahimsa in action.

As with all the yamas, ahimsa is completely subjective, and what is right and nonviolent for you isn't necessarily the prescription to live by for another. There is an element of ahimsa, however, that is rarely spoken about, which is fundamental to so much human suffering and attachment—nonviolence towards ourselves. While we are busting a gut to step over ants and eat cruelty free products, we are self-criticising, self-hating, self-harming and running a 24/7 negative soundtrack inside our heads.

In workshops and Q & A sessions, I spend a lot of time calling people out on questions that start with 'This is a dumb question', which of course is code for 'I am dumb'. It lodges like a shard of glass every time I hear the implicit self-deprecation used to demean and diminish out of the mouths of people who are walking around in a miasma of internal loathing.

In one session I had a student asking me about building a personal brand—she was concerned that no one would come to her yoga classes when she graduated from her teacher training because, as she put it, she 'has such a boring and ordinary name'. She wanted to know if she should change her name? She so obviously saw herself as invisible and forgettable, and assumed that this was the world's experience of her too. That is a perfect example of violence by stealth. We are so used to hearing our own inner critic that we don't have an awareness of the damage we are doing to ourselves.

I mentioned earlier the personal struggle I had with not feeling good enough, and the resulting need to overachieve. I remember lying in bed the night I was awarded my PhD and sobbing into my pillow. I'd achieved the highest possible academic qualification I could get, and I'd completed it in under three years while working in a demanding executive role. It should have been an occasion to celebrate the heights of what can be done with hard work, discipline and willpower, but instead, it brought the startling realisation that I still felt unworthy and unfulfilled. (That's Dr Unworthy to you.)

Happily, the absurdity of this behaviour was a moment that truly rang alarm bells for me. It forced me to turn in and start the process of making peace with my samvega, to look for a happiness that wasn't based on thankless striving and craving approval from some external authority. Ahimsa begins at home, and before you can good hustle for others, there has to be self-love and compassion.

New business endeavours and making the leap into pursuing your dharma can be fraught with brutal criticism. There are standard limiting beliefs that I see and hear so often—the most common is that no one would be interested in what the business is going to do or say or sell. Of course that attitude is also underpinned by the familiar adversary of unworthiness—which is strongly linked to comparison and judgement. If you are posing the question 'Why me?', you are simultaneously asking 'Why not them?' and comparing yourself to a faceless competitor that embodies all of the attributes you believe you lack. Before you have even committed your idea to paper or screen you are writing it off, handing over your power and prowess to something or someone who doesn't even exist. It's madness, but it's a common madness. With that level of self-doubt, the first naysayer you share your idea with is enough to send you scurrying back into your negative belief system.

ii) Satya

Which leads us into the second yama—satya, or truth. You need to make a commitment to yourself to not only not harm, but to also tell the truth. In her excellent book *Fierce Medicine*, yoga teacher Ana Forrest devotes a whole chapter to what she calls 'truth speaking'. Forrest defines this as speaking from the heart, and telling the truth—with compassion. Many of us have lost the art of truth speaking. I'm not suggesting that we are lying our way though our days and nights, but rather that we have so much fear and so many filters, that we look to say what we want people to hear, rather than what would be the kind or compassionate thing to say to them. Truth speaking asks us to firstly open our hearts. There needs to be some preparatory work beforehand to ensure that our heart once open is resilient. We need to know, trust and love ourselves before our truth speaking, as we also have to be able to hear it from others. If you have an active self-critic and a dry reservoir of self-love, you can't pour onto another what you aren't able to give or receive yourself.

All too often words are used as weapons. It takes time and discipline to turn that pattern off. We are cruel with words to be funny, to be defensive, to be liked and approved of, to lash out or back, or simply because we lack awareness and compassion. Truth speaking has to have a trifold target of ourselves, the person we are speaking to, and the situation, and all need compassion within them. There are many times that the best truth speaking is silently witnessing someone else's pain with love and empathy, and not giving them the benefit of your wisdom. These are the times when the truth is that they have to work through their own stuff. Your power is in compassion and simply being present and honouring what they are going through. This is a beautiful yogic practice, and actively seeking opportunities to listen without judgement is an abundant training ground.

Truth speaking for justice is a much-needed intervention, and is often a frightening exposure to power and the force of public or majority opinion. As a good hustler, this will be a lightning rod for you, as your practice will be based on working and sometimes fighting for something that is bigger than you, for the greater good of humanity. Sure, this is subjective, and whenever there is a division of public sentiment on a matter, there is an equally passionate argument from the opposing side as to why they are right. Hello wars. Truth speaking here is not about winning the argument or hating the opposition, it is about standing up for what you believe in. That may be just a matter of not letting a sexist, racist, discriminatory or unkind comment pass without asking the speaker not to make those comments in front of you, as you find them offensive.

We often choose to stay silent because it is easier, or we don't want to become the target ourselves. Or we are frightened that it might impact our careers, or what people think and say about us. And the answer is yes, it might. By voicing your truth in a compassionate way, you are acknowledging the speaker, the victim and your own truth. Whether or not the acid is turned on you is irrelevant. Your path to enlightenment, or even a good night's sleep and a clear conscience, must have truth in its DNA.

It is about the broader commitment to humanity and your own commitment to living as your perfect and divine self.

A good hustle is built on the scaffolds of self-awareness, and it's usually pretty clear when you need to speak up. You can feel that voice welling in your gut, dying to burst out if it can only get past the fear filter in your throat. Satya in creating your good hustle is of premium importance as, like with all relationships, complexities escalate quickly when there is money and risk at stake. By not identifying when you are uncomfortable with a proposal, or the ethics or motives of someone you are dealing with, you are silencing that inner compass that you are working so hard to polish and give a voice to.

When starting a new business, everyone is an expert, and you'll get a truckload of advice along the way. This isn't a bad thing, as the early conversations, especially the ones with potential customers, are essential for refining what you are doing. What you may find in many conversations, and be surprised by, are the strong voices of criticism, doom, gloom and caution. Unless what you are doing is truly high risk—not just to you but to others—and the concern is genuine truth speaking (you know, mortgaging the house again for a highly speculative Ponzi scheme), then often the truth coming your way arises from the speaker's own fear or previous life experience, or a desire but inability to do exactly what you are doing.

Be wary of your reaction to these conversations, and always listen for your own truth. There is a point in the process where you must just begin. Assuming you are conducting your own risk management and due diligence, and putting your idea through its paces before you bet everything on black, the combination of knowledge and skills, plus heart and gut, should give you all of the answers you need. If you believe there is no clear and present danger and that the benefits to you of having a go, even if you fail, are more compelling than where you are currently at, then nothing should hold you back. If you're continually getting advice that there is a flaw in your business model, but you believe you can overcome it and push on, then you are making and owning that decision, and it is part of your karma. Ultimately, whatever the outcome, you will have actively chosen the journey.

iii) Asteya

The third precept of the yamas, asteya, or non-stealing, seems a little more cut and dried—or is it? Stealing can be material; beyond the material, however—especially in relation to the journey of our good hustles from idea to reality—we can apply asteya to a number of key points along the way. It is often said that there is nothing new in the world, inferring that we live in a space of continual reinvention, solving and improving on the eternal and repetitive problems of humanity. This suggests that there are few opportunities to truly come up with an idea for something that is unique. The definition of innovation is bringing something new and transformational to an existing idea, and in the main this is what we build on with new ideas. When you bring your new idea into the light of day, you have a responsibility to ensure that you aren't inadvertently infringing on the rights of any existing products, services or brands. This is easily done with the power of a search engine, or the use of trained professionals in the case of checking for brand and trade infringements or patent searches.

It may well be that someone else is doing exactly what you want to do, but your innovation is that it is new to your area, jurisdiction or country. All good, no theft there. It may well be that you can reach out to whomever is doing what you want to do and get their help and advice as you start your own journey; never underestimate the power of entrepreneurs to support others.

It is quite common, in the excitement of beginning to turn your idea into a business, to inadvertently ignore or overlook this yama. I'm as guilty as the next person of doing little projects 'off the side of my desk' and never really thinking about who is paying for my side hustle. When I worked in large government departments and well-funded universities, this seemed to be okay, and I had almost a sense of entitlement. I believed that the hard work and endless sweat I put into my job had earned me some invisible credits that allowed me to clock on to my own work every so often, and maybe even do a little printing. I know, right—it's trivial and we all do it. But that isn't the point. When the yogi antenna is tuned well, this is stealing, no matter how we might like to justify it, and we need to be mindful, and apply some satya to the justification.

You can see how even small acts are part of the fabric of ethics and right living. The point isn't who knows or cares, the point is that we know and care and say no. In your quest to get your good hustle on, consider how that might work for you. Maybe the first step, if you are nervous about leaping into starting a business, is to approach your employer and see how they feel about enabling some creative time for employees. Some businesses, following the lead of companies like Google and Pixar, allow a regular allotment of time for employees to undertake their own projects every week. Look for opportunities to try out the signs you are on your dharma path without taking away from what you are being paid to do. Want to teach yoga? Great—offer to run lunchtime classes for your stressed-out workmates in the boardroom in exchange for a gold coin donation to charity. Want to work in organics or run a food truck? Too easy—get approval to have some urban food gardens set up within your offices, or set up a lunchtime food supply for co-workers to raise money for office social activities or charity. Love crafting and dream of a social enterprise? Organise a meet-up with your co-workers and see how many of them are avid knitters, spinners or scrapbookers who have been yearning for a peer group and you will have just provided one—with an on-site Christmas makers' market opportunity for all of your gorgeous outputs to be sold.

Another area where you can easily become guilty of inadvertent stealing is when seeking advice from other people. All of us tend to indulge in it when we are at the low-cash/high-need part of our business idea development. I'm asked nearly every day to have coffee with someone so they can run something past me or 'pick my brain'. I used to think that it was part of my karma yoga to meet up and have these conversations. But it didn't take long to realise that this was really cutting into my own work time.

The answer was solved with love, compassion and clear boundaries. I stopped having coffee and instead I now offer to review an idea pitch by email and give some advice on the next steps, ensuring I give value and let them know what the costs of the next steps are. It also enables them to understand that they have to invest in their ideas from the beginning. And I say no a lot, too. I also allocate an amount of time to pro-bono work with social enterprises, not-for-profits, or brilliant good hustle ideas that I want to play with. When asking others for help—especially those who do it for a living—remember that everyone has a value and if you need to ask for it for free, then make a loving gesture of acknowledgement to say thank you.

The final area where you may need to look at how you can use the yama of asteya is linked to the same way ahimsa is applied to self-harm. What emotional patterns are you getting stuck in or hanging on to that are robbing you of happiness? Is it anxiety? Is it fear? Is it jealousy? It is shame and regret? Is it pride and reputational attachment? All of these feelings steal joy and keep you stuck in the past or terrified of the future, rather than settled, at peace and at one in the present. Think about where you can put asteya to work in your life and make a commitment to focus on that area in your meditation, yoga and mind management. Root out the cause and the effect from your mind and on your life. Bring these feelings into your meditation and yoga and work through them on the mat and on the cushion. Stop resisting them and embrace them as part of you with the disarmament of self-love and compassion. This is theft that is not just daylight but 24/7 robbery, and only you can apprehend the offender.

iv) Brahmacharya

The fourth yama is always a beauty to discuss. Guaranteed to elicit awkward shoe staring or (if you're like me) immature giggling and juvenile comments. Brahmacharya, or chastity, is a great example of how social shifts from Patanjali's time to the modern context change the intention of the ashtanga yoga system in word, if not in deed. Chastity was a given if you were going to be a renunciate yogi, and still is for the *sanyasins, babas,* sadhus, monks, *bhikkhus* and nuns who take on a holistic commitment to their spiritual path. In Sanskrit, 'Brahma' means 'higher awareness' and 'acharya' means 'to live in'. Brahmacharya therefore means to move, learn and live in higher awareness. For the stricter religious and non-sectarian definition, brahmacharya means complete control over or abstinence from sexual interactions. I believe that there is a compatibility, however, with contemporary practice. Like the divine itself, there are many ways to incorporate and understand brahmacharya in the spirit of living in higher awareness. In the Buddhist monastic tradition, celibacy is a method of dealing with desire. In his book *Work, Sex, Money: Real Life on the Path of Mindfulness*, Chögyam Trungpa describes celibacy as not designed to repress desire, but to 'examine the mental aspect of it'. He goes on to explain that physical expression is an extension of mental desire, so sort out the mind and the body will follow. Once the desire is understood, the heat goes out of it as something that can distract and derail your mind from what you are trying to achieve. Monastics are using their sexual energy for spiritual purposes. In the period of aligning your mind, instilling discipline and focusing on your business idea, this is an option as part of repurposing your energies into the single-pointed goal of your good hustle. If you aren't quite ready to get *that* serious about your business (remember, I am a method yogi), I think the idea of brahmacharya is worth considering in a world that is gorging itself on sexualised images and low self-esteem.

The way I see brahmacharya in our context feeds entirely and logically into the progression from nonviolence, to truth, to non-stealing. Sex outside of committed loving relationships is frequently used as a gateway activity to the future promise of love or simply as a way of receiving attention and approval. Let me be perfectly clear that I'm not implying that sex outside of marriage or relationships is a bad thing. Decades of feminist fighting for the right to have pleasure on our terms has been a good thing. The collective eroding of women's self-esteem that seems to have quietly happened alongside increased sexual freedom, however, means that sex can be an agent of violence and theft, and benefits enormously from being reframed against Patanjali's eight limbs. Approaching this from a Buddhist perspective on attachment and non-attachment is another way to think about your relationship to sex, and thus its impact on your mind and emotions.

You can ask yourself the question: does or will engaging in sex at this time with this being cause me suffering?

The idea of attachment here is not whether the act causes you physical pain (see your doctor, m'kay!) but whether the emotions, reactions and expectations of sex or love leave you with an attachment or craving or aversion that causes suffering. The answer may be no; that you can, within or outside of a loving relationship, have sexual interactions that leave you neither attached to the pleasure nor suffering in any way. I think we have established that before you can get down to business, you need to attend to the discipline of mind, and surrender, and acceptance of your own perfection, exactly as you are right now. The search for love from an external other is a big distraction, and can significantly derail the real search for love that is undertaken within. No matter how fantastic a partner appears, without mind control and self-love conquered on your side, that other person is going to have to go through it all with you, and potentially be the recipient of a lot of acting out as you grow. Now maybe that's okay, and part of their karmic path with you and for themselves. But it also may be better to turn your love light down, and get down to the business of working on your mind, so when the divine comes knocking, you are ready to entertain.

v) Aparigraha

We end the yamas with aparigraha, which translates in a number of ways including 'non-greed', 'non-possessiveness', and 'non-attachment'. The prefix 'a' means 'non', 'pari' means 'on all sides', and the word 'graha' means to take, to seize, or to grab. This important yama teaches us to take only what we need, keep only what serves us in the moment, and to let go when the time is right. For entrepreneurs it reminds us that our endeavours only have to yield enough. That the game is actually about working towards something that provides service and benefit, while covering our needs and contributing to the wellbeing of others. We don't need to hustle to accrue, we simply need to be sustainable and conscious.

Aparigraha is actually one of the central messages in the Bhagavad Gita, in which Krishna shares with Arjuna one of the teachings that could perhaps be the most important lesson of all to learn: *'Let your concern be with action alone, and never with the fruits of action. Do not let the results of action be your motive.'* How often do we worry so much about what might come of the effort we put into a project at work, that we never really enjoy the work itself? So often we worry if we'll be successful enough, or good enough when we put our hearts on the line to show the world what we're made of, that we forget why we started in the first place. The essential point here is that we should never concern ourselves with the outcome of a situation, we should only concern ourselves with what we're actually doing right now as we work towards that outcome. Staying present and in the moment is fundamental to the ashtanga yoga system.

The end of the yamas and the beginning of the niyamas is asking us to release control while knowing that we have a very clear set of moral guidelines that can be applied as a template to what we do and how we do it. Does whatever it is you are interrogating in your life currently fit within that paradigm? If so, surrender and proceed with yogi abandon.

2. The Niyamas

Niyama, the second limb of ashtanga, means observances; these are recommended activities and habits for healthy living, spiritual enlightenment and a liberated state of existence. The niyamas tend to be activities that are more turned inwards; they are self-reflective tools that allow us to deepen our understanding of the yogic path and our place on it. Their focus is being rather than doing. As the yamas and niyamas are some of the building blocks of your yogic practice, it is essential that they are part of the integrated thinking of how you approach things, rather than you seeing your spiritual life as separate from your greater living and working.

Like the yamas, there are five niyamas or observances to master in your yogi skill set. I'm again going to link them to the process of thinking about your good hustle. They are: 'saucha' (cleanliness), 'santosha' (contentment), 'tapas' (austerity), 'svadhaya' (self study) and 'ishvara pranidhana' (union with the divine).

i) Saucha

The niyamas begin with saucha or cleanliness, which can be applied in a literal approach, as regular bathing and keeping your surroundings clean and tidy. It can also be used metaphorically in terms of the state of your mind and actions. Undoubtedly, personal hygiene was of utmost importance to yogis and householders, and featured in the daily pre- and post-prayer and meditation ritual. It was seen as a mark of respect and worship.

The split between saucha as both metaphorical and applied remains relevant to our contemporary practice. I would hazard that we are frantically sanitising our surfaces and fighting against germs because our minds are so full of compost, and it is easier to work with what is outside than get into our innermost trash and do the difficult work. There is, as yet, no wipe invented that can do the work of sanitising the mind. It is our minds that need to be tamed, cleaned of their grasping and attachment to sense pleasures, and then situated in the present. Think of your mind as a work surface. If you are struggling to find space with piles of mess around you, it is going to be much harder to sit down and focus on the task at hand.

As we are preparing for understanding our path and working on our good hustle concepts, the process of getting a stable and clean workspace is a daily task. As with any big clean-up, it is hideous at first. It feels overwhelming, and with every piece of junk you throw out, you discover hidden repositories of new rubbish to deal with. It is a tough visceral process that makes you want to simply shut the door and leave it for another time. The tip for pushing on is to continually chip away at the pile. Remember you have the control over this process, and you own all the crap. The classic hallmark of hoarders is the inability to emotionally release all of their possessions. The mess ends up owning you, and therefore it is incumbent on you to shift the power paradigm and get back on top. You're the boss.

The anatomy of a thought, a pattern, an emotional response is an interesting concept. It is hard for us to initially conceive that feelings and thoughts are habits, not reality. We feel something once, in a particular set of circumstances. Let's say someone is nice to us, we then feel good when we next see that person, as we associate them with not feeling bad. That nice feeling was previously learned when we encountered it in a positive situation, and so on and so on. The feeling is not a thing within itself. We think feelings are real, and we think they come from the body. They aren't, and they don't, they are simply an artefact of our minds. We make them, and we can change them.

We store events and our reactions to them in our emotional sponge like a repository to keep amplifying and morphing the good and the bad into their distinct categories. Even the act of cleaning out your mind gets a tag attached, most likely bad, so you are resisting and reacting even before you get to the act of doing.

But what if you approached these mind messes as simply neutral? Not good, not bad, a task to be done, which if fully present in the moment simply involves some conscious dismissing of thoughts when they pop up. Suddenly, the work of saucha is manageable and in fact becomes a routine that is undertaken quickly and efficiently when spills occur. Before you know it, what felt like an enormous archive of waste is a neatly ordered file that fits comfortably anywhere, making you nimble and agile, so as to cleanly address whatever undertaking you are considering. Saucha is both mindfulness *and* meditation.

Perhaps you need to undertake some regular meditation sessions to hone your ability to identify when you are about to get caught up in a thought that will catch you in a quicksand of mess. As mentioned before, once you have learned these new neural responses, you will instantly flip into mind maintenance mode and not get buried in a hoarder's paradise.

ii) Santosha

After the effort and intensity of undertaking the process of saucha, the next niyama is the far gentler santosha, or contentment. On the journey to enlightenment, escape from the distraction of material pleasures feels like a safe and still harbour. If ever there was a benchmark for being present, it is santosha, as contentment indicates that right here, right now, all is well. Contentment can't be parsed in the idea that you will be content once you acquire something else, or achieve another goal. I believe contentment is the best indicator that you are working through the eight limbs and assimilating the learnings, as wherever there is yearning or discontent, there is residual attachment, and clearly you are yet to completely release yourself from the idea that external things and achievements are defining you and your happiness.

Contentment in your good hustle sits in the knowing that you are living in dharma. Santosha in your good hustle building blocks comes from knowing that you have a limited view of what is possible. And within the narrow confines of experience and imagination, there is a vast repertoire of alternative outcomes, events and endings. So living in your dharma means you follow the sense where you are most in flow.

In this mindset of santosha, when your good hustle ideas meet with a curveball or roadblock there is a deep mental and physical sense of wellbeing because you know that whatever is happening is right. The redirect is just a recalibration of your worldview into a new way of thinking and being. You're not attached to what you thought was going to happen, as you know that you could only see a fraction of the possibilities. Achieving santosha is a function of learning how to be happy with whatever is. A super easy statement to make, but as with everything in the eight limbs, it requires a constant and dedicated process of awareness and discipline around what is real, and what is unreal. Where we have given value, meaning and power to material things, which are by their nature impermanent, this is the unreal. Where happiness comes from people, sensations or experiences, which are by their nature impermanent, this is the unreal. Only change and impermanence are real. It is a constant vigilance that our minds don't sneak back to their habitual patterns. Consider this in relation to good hustle; especially if you are at the ideation stage, everything is going to seem pretty unreal, and most of what you know will be based only on perception. This is where agility comes in. When everything is impermanent it is easy to rapidly change, as it is essentially what you expect to do.

This isn't to say that happiness and other sensations and situations can't be experienced. The subtle difference is the understanding that happiness doesn't come from expectations about objects or experiences. It comes from a sense of connection, of oneness and of, ultimately, santosha. As soon as you start classifying objects and experiences, including people, into categories of 'good' or 'bad', 'happy' or 'sad', you are creating an imaginary subjectivity where you cling to one and push away from the other. Both of which create attachment and thus suffering. The project is to experience everything without the swings, the highs and lows, simply with surrender, and contentment. This seems impossible, doesn't it? Our minds are so conditioned to constantly judge and classify everything and everyone, accepting and rejecting, reifying or demonising, working away as if we are in charge of and responsible for it all. Which in itself is exhausting; no wonder we are increasingly anxious and reactive, and far away from santosha so much of the time. Santosha may well be a distinct niyama; however, it is also a checkpoint. When santosha is present and constant in our lives, we have achieved the preconditions for adapting to the remaining niyamas.

iii) Tapas

Which brings us to tapas, or austerities. For most new businesses, the pathway from idea to market is a period of time where money is going out far more quickly than it is coming in. Some of that money will be spent on research and development, testing markets, trying different angles in advertising and marketing, and making prototypes. This is expenditure where the return on investment is not a boomerang. It is also completely normal. The majority of businesses, even if they have a short pathway between concept and sale, are revenue negative or neutral at the outset. Planning and budgeting for this period of time through exercising some austerities definitely makes it easier to keep the dream alive without falling into the chasm of worry and concern that comes with the early part of venture creation.

Our Western understanding of austerities and suffering simply doesn't allow these definitions to be anything but pejorative. We live in a state where our whole existence is geared towards the acquisition of material goods, sense enjoyment and emotional comfort. The idea that austerity is a choice, and can be highly beneficial to our quest for happiness or contentment, is anathema to our understanding of existence.

Austerities in yoga and in the good hustle are what could be described as blessings in disguise. I'd go so far to say that they don't even require a disguise, they are blatant advantages. By being able to release attachment to sense pleasures and go without, you are able to clearly see the real from the unreal, and let go of what doesn't serve you. In the Yoga Sutras, tapas, like saucha, can be both physical and mental. Captured in the type of austerities practised by yogis are material things like restriction on food (quantity and type), on comfort more generally (warmth and soft beds), and on actions and interactions of the mind (such as thoughts and behaviours).

Throughout this book is the (possibly maddening by now) mantra that meditation and mind management are the gateway activities to happiness. If you are at the starting blocks without an existing practice, and let's assume we are all still happily (or unhappily) wallowing in lives rich with samsara, some austerities are necessary. Undertaking austerities is the initial pathway to neural reprogramming. Getting out of your cosy bed in the dark of morning to meditate is an austerity. You are giving up warmth and sleep to sit still, breathe, concentrate and develop the mental discipline necessary. And it doesn't end there. If you are like me, with a love of (read: shocking attachment to) food, and your life revolves around planning and executing delicious meals, it is an absolute austerity measure to shift from food as entertainment, status, pleasure and companion to it being fuel for the body. AUSTERITY ALERT. Add into the mix prohibitions on killing and violence, as required in the first yama ahimsa, and you are also saying goodbye to eating animals and fish and, depending on your level of dedication, eggs and dairy, too. Oh, and then there's alcohol, variously a stimulant or intoxicant, and not a feature of the yogic lifestyle. There is a continuum of shock and naaaaaaaw that many of us feel at the thought of giving up these parts of our cultural practices, which seem so essentially human; and so necessary to fit into our various groups and tribes, most of which have eating and drinking at their celebratory centre. Our collective cultural obsession with food is bordering on obscene, yet we rarely question the reason that eating and entertaining is our new place of worship.

All this digestive attachment and grasping is considered a significant impediment to spiritual practice. Here the difficulty of austerity is wildly amplified because we have such a tsunami of enjoyment to constantly decline. At the point where you are ready, you may find, as I did, that what once seemed to be the most difficult or impossible task simply feels right, and you begin the process of decoupling from your food affair. What was once an austerity becomes the new normal, as does getting up early, feeling compassion for the greater mass of humans in all their complexity, and looking beyond the needs of one to the needs of all. When your mind and body aren't consumed by consuming, there is much more space to devote to good hustling. In many spiritual traditions fasting is a regular part of practice to bring clarity and concentration for meditation, and food reduction or at least mindfulness is a great habit to get into.

This is where the practice of tapas needs some good PR. We need to embrace and seek out opportunities to exercise our discipline muscles. Saying no to the things that distract us, and at worst derail us, is a choice to be celebrated. Initially you have to move through the pain of letting go. Once we have deprogrammed the addiction behaviour, we begin to experience the calm and constant feeling of deep contentment.

The long-term adoption of austerities has many benefits aside from enhanced spiritual capacity. There are significant savings to be made by not indulging ourselves every time we slip from sensory euphoria into the depression of non-gratification. Add it up. Drinking, partying, shopping—it all costs money. Productivity gains go through the roof. Waking up every day feeling fresh and full of juice is incredible, and that enjoyment doesn't diminish. When you have awareness about consumption as a panacea for suffering, you make better choices about what you really need.

Our bodies get better with yoga or any kind of regular physical practice. Our minds get better with regular meditation. Together with removing the rubbish from our bodies and our habits, and building our mind muscles, what was an austerity becomes like a jackpot. We've just switched up our worldview. Suddenly month-long retreats, upping our hours on the yoga mat or meditation cushion, and giving up those residual dietary treats don't seem like an extreme sport. They seem desirable. And right about here, the place where we couldn't possibly give up our jobs, take a pay cut and risk everything to follow the dream of our dharma, suddenly seems to be achievable. We are no longer slaves to desire and attachment, we are the bosses of our own minds. This is the point at which it all makes sense, and the words about self-discipline and doing the mind work that were empty and academic become the point of transition. It is more than talk about journeys or steps along a path. It is an embodied and emboldened lived experience, with real, tangible benefits not dependant on something outside of us.

This is a moment of realisation we need to savour, as it is a significant point of acknowledgement of how much we are the authors of our own happiness and suffering.

Let me note again, this isn't about creating a life without comfort or ease, far from it. It is about navigating through an awareness of how much we sleepwalk through life with the soporific effects of our favourite distractions and numbing tools constantly at hand. Austerities are essential when re-prioritising your life to get you to a place of living in dharma, and they definitely can't make you feel like you are in lack or in loss. They should feel empowering and driven by choice.

Austerities at this point in time in your good hustle can be about finding ways to save and minimise expenditure so you have a comfortable buffer. You need to be able to withstand any unplanned blowouts that might (actually, definitely) will happen. The austerities you go through will also be personal. If you are working another job, and building your good hustle dream around the fringes of the day, you may find you have little free time, as every moment will be taken up with nibbling away at your goals. Especially while managing family and life and keeping up spiritual practices. Sleep can be sacrificed and is a small price to pay for being able to carve out a couple of precious extra hours in a day. You need to adopt a single-pointed approach to the world. At every opportunity, ask yourself if what you are about to do gets you closer to your goal.

Once you have landed on your business idea and have mapped out a tentative pathway to get your idea to market, you will be faced with daily distractions and decisions. I've seen it happen over and over again. When the light of creativity and entrepreneurialism is switched on, suddenly the tsunami of opportunities flows in and your simple idea becomes the generator of many, many new tangents. I like to call this dilemma 'opportun-itis', and it is a disease that can be terminal to a project if left untreated. This is not to say that any of the new twists and turns you've thought of wouldn't be successful, but the reality is that you have to start somewhere, and execute that idea, before adding in all the bells and whistles. Resources, especially your own capacity, are finite, and you need to be absolutely ruthless about what you will allow to use up your precious time, money and energy. Austerities are also about knowing when to say no to losing focus; the answer is to call on the Yoga Sutras and limit your opportun-itis with tapas.

By getting comfortable with austerities as a necessary part of your good hustle practice, you gain a simple way to keep on track. By relating everything you do to what you're trying to achieve, decisions are unambiguous. It's a strategy deployed by everyone from entrepreneurs to athletes to get where they need to go, as suddenly everything that doesn't serve them falls away.

Buddhist teacher Lama Zopa Rinpoche says that every morning, the first thought of the day should be setting an intention that all activities undertaken should work solely towards the liberation of all sentient beings from suffering. Any action can be decided by that simple tenet alone. Aside from being a pretty good way to start the day, this question, or something like it, can supplement your good hustle decision-making template. Does the action move you further towards your goal, and does it equally give opportunities to serve others with unconditional love? When these are the underpinnings, it's hard to see how austerities can possibly be a bad thing. When it comes to expenses, the same strategy can be applied—will the purchase essentially contribute to your next goal in getting to live in your dharma? If no, then it's a clear and simple decision that can be made without any compromise or heeding of your needy inner voice.

iv) Svadhaya

The penultimate niyama is svadhaya, or the study of the self. As with the previous niyamas, this can be both a literal and a metaphoric experience. To really understand the complexities of the mind, time has to be spent interrogating thoughts and sitting with the processes that go on unchecked within us. Here's the thing. Everything in our mental consciousness is a conceptual story, our own opinion. Everything. And what's worse, our consciousness is a liar. Neuroses are 'I' based. Based on layers of lies. You know this junk, it's what we've been talking about for chapters; keep reminding yourself that none of it is true, it's just opinion that flows down the river of your thoughts. Svadhaya takes us on a trip down that river. Paddling along with intent, able to veer down a tributary if necessary, cataloging all of the varieties of plants, animals and litter we find above, below and alongside our mind canoes.

Unsurprisingly, meditation is the vehicle that allows this to unfold, and as the preceding niyamas are undertaken, the way is cleared for practice to get deeper, for insights to occur and for revelations to lead to further renunciation. All of the niyamas build resilience and awakening to the true nature of self. Our attachments, our conditioning and entanglement with the desire for permanence means that it takes space and time to get to the point where real self-study can occur. Much of the work in saucha is demolishing the mess of our minds, cleaning up the illusions, and leaving the good bones of our mental structure to work with. As we become more familiar with what and who we are, and more interconnected with our compassionate relationship with others, the ability comes to sit less in the ego 'I' and more in the greater community of humanity. We are the observer not the doer in our thoughts.

The capacity to take the role of observer is important in self-study as we have to be able to observe our behaviour in an impartial way. This can, at the outset of our meditation practice, be like an ongoing dialogue with ourselves as we document the goings-on of our mind. There I am craving chocolate, there I am judging another, there I am judging myself, there I am full of the pride of doing meditation, there I am believing I'm a better/worse person, there I am making up stories about my life, there I am believing my lying consciousness. And on it goes. By noting and dismissing these thoughts, we see the patterns and subtly redirect, calling ourselves out on our habitual critic in the process. In doing so we are building new ways of thinking, where we strongly acknowledge that the old pattern of thinking isn't serving us. After a period of time, we begin to autocorrect even as the thought starts to form, self-censoring the behaviour that pushes us back into a fear-based egoic loop of clinging and criticism. Once this new voice becomes established, the real progress of fighting against the ideas and emotional patterns that keep us fettered begins in earnest.

I see this as distinctly different from a practice of relentless positivity and affirmation where perceived negativity isn't countenanced for fear that it will somehow stain the rainbow. By observing all our thoughts without apportioning them as good or bad, our totality is the subject of self-study. There is no annex of fear, self-hate and negativity being pushed back by positivity until it spectacularly breaks out at the most inconvenient time. And this is where we can really know ourselves, our whole selves. We aren't being self-critical or self-loathing, we are just integrating and acknowledging who we are, while building the mind towards who we want to be. No part of us is left behind, there is no shadow self, as all of us is available, and welcome.

At the same time as we conduct our self-study, we can study texts and consult teachers that are going to grow our wisdom. This is the duality of svadhaya where the self-study is both internal and a process of wisdom acquisition. Accessing along the way teachers who help you reach your goals is an important part of your growth. Reading this book and texts like it is an element of that. In many Eastern belief systems, it is understood that we are born with our own divine wisdom fully installed. It is the samsara experienced through living in the world that confuses and distracts us from the ultimate work of living our dharma. You could say we are finding our way back to us, with reminders along the way, like a treasure hunt where the clues are too quiet to hear over the noise of sense pleasures.

Our teachers on the path to self-study appear in many guises, and often unpredictably. Most of us will have had a teacher at school who somehow cut through and saw who we were. They lit a spark in us of self-belief that helped to wipe away a little of the dirt obscuring our view. Some of our teachers in life are painful and difficult to hold in our memories with compassion and grace. But we must. These teachers appear all through our lives, and the closer attention we pay to our svadhaya, the more we are able to listen to the teachings. Don't be tempted to see hardship and pain as roadblocks. See them as some ripened karma that, once cleared, will deliver great virtue. Resist the temptation to run to a safe, comfortable spot; combat the rising aversion with patience and fortitude, knowing it will pass.

In the West we have been undoubtedly jaded in the way we view spiritual teachers or 'gurus', many of whom have been presented to us as exotic figures from the East. We often follow with little discrimination only to later find they are revealed as charlatans and fakes—or, more accurately, people just like us. The guru in many spiritual traditions plays the role of a teacher and leader, they take us with confidence and rigour into our next levels of discovery, especially in unravelling complex spiritual texts like the ones we are working with here. It is only because of the many, many interpretations and commentaries available to us that we are able to understand what those enlightened sages were trying to tell us all those centuries ago. One person's guru is another's charlatan, however, which is why it is important to read, follow, listen to, challenge, criticise and observe the teachers and their teachings that resonate most with you. They are awakening in you your own wisdom.

My advice in matters of self-study and the pursuit of knowledge is to cast your net wide. Go down a lot of unmarked streets, and constantly be vigilant about what your mind is telling you. If a book jumps off a shelf at you, read it—even if the author is someone you never would have considered to be speaking your language. Where opportunities present, say yes, and with an open but critical mind listen and learn. You will undoubtedly hit the paydirt of resonation at the end of a meandering ramble that you didn't think was leading anywhere special or spiritual.

Especially when on that nervous, excited cusp of starting something new, the temptation is to wallow in endless learning. Women are repeat offenders in believing that they need more and more knowledge to be able to successfully execute a business idea. You have to look out for the point at which the quest for knowledge becomes a safe haven for doing nothing and avoiding wisdom. No book or teacher is ever going to be able to teach you precisely how to do what it is that you are trying to achieve. Until you have actually gone out and begun yourself, you will not be actualising your learning, merely stockpiling. When all the books are read, podcasts are listened to, blogs are scanned and tweets and posts consumed, there is a point at which you have to rely on your own wisdom and begin.

You'll be surprised at how authoritative you actually are, and how empowering it is to get started and make some decisions. As long as you are open to things not always being as you imagined, before long you will realise you are capably *doing* business. Even if you are still feeling the remnants of thinking you are merely an actor playing a role, these are only the opinions of your mind. That you are doing it is living proof of your competency. The process of self-study continues in parallel with life. It, too, is a practice, and needs to be a diligent one as you integrate your work and what it teaches you with your own svadhaya.

v) Ishvara Pranidhana

At the end of it all is ishvara pranidhana, surrender to the divine. This whole process has been a continuum leading to your own preparedness to meet that part of you, or your belief system, that offers you unconditional love, entirely reliant on nothing but you. There is a common belief that enlightenment, once reached, is like a void or a blank of space and silence; that the enlightened disappear into another realm leaving nothing behind. Lama Zopa Rinpoche argues that it is the opposite—it is exactly like life is right now, with a sense of unshakeable, inconceivable equanimity, of blissful interconnectedness. The purpose behind the search for enlightenment isn't to remove yourself from the world you have spent so long and worked so hard to integrate into. It is to be fully alive and awake to the miracle of you, and us, and everything in the world. As you work towards finding your way to that place, the restraints and observances of the yamas and niyamas are there to guide, prepare and upskill you to reach the divinity within. I don't believe that liberation, or enlightenment, is a moment of excessive fanfare and fireworks. I believe it is found in the absence of creating suffering; in the moment when you haven't reacted to a situation of immense stress, where you have felt limitless love and compassion for those who do you both good and ill; where your action and your heart meet and merge.

I think we are given glimpses of ishvara pranidhana, tastes that nourish and encourage us to keep going, until those morsels add up to a greater and greater amount of time where your mind is content. Attachment is replaced by the genuine desire for all beings to be happy and free. At this point, you bring that essence to whatever business or project you are undertaking. Then everything that you turn your hands, mind and heart to delivers dharma. It's not in the doing after all, it's in the being. You will naturally embody this state. In your work you will model this, and inspire others to have what you're having. This will draw to you the community that supports you and values the way you want to live your life. You will be doing what you love, because you will love everything. In your good hustle, ishvara pranidhana is best described as the point at which you find that thing you know, without doubt, is your dharma. It is where your yearning for your true nature of self, and the clear vision of what it is you are capable of doing, is clearly revealed.

Business on the Path to Enlightenment

The yamas and niyamas, as two laundry lists of activities, are themselves a fair undertaking, but both are essential in progressing along the path of becoming a contemporary, good hustling yogi, of being able to create heart-centred businesses that are ripe with meaning and resilient. The heavy lifting is done at the front end, with constant ongoing maintenance required to ensure that the evolution in your way of being continues. It can feel like the yamas and niyamas alone are sufficient for Patanjali to have stopped there. It is a lifelong process.

So, too, is the developing of a new business idea.

It is this work of creativity, ideation, untrammelled thinking and unlimited wonder that takes you through all of the potentials and allows you to narrow them down through a process of logical and intuitive elimination. The destination is the place where you don't want to look for anything else. It has to be something that is big enough to make a difference but small enough to be able to manage to bring it to life. It must contain the elements of compassion and love that make it the project that will allow you to feel like you have arrived in your life as an active participant, not a dupe hanging on the strings of someone else's responsibility.

3. Asana

Now the twin peaks of the yamas and niyamas are climbed, we turn to the next arm of Patanjali's eight limbs. Asanas are the postures practised in yoga, the physical activity that the majority of people in the West recognise as yoga. Asana needs to be put in the context of where yoga came from, and what it was designed to do, to help you to understand where it fits in your good hustle. In India, asana was a practice to gain flexibility and strength to prepare the body for long hours of sitting in meditation. Yoga was principally undertaken by men. This is in strong contrast to how it has been adopted in the West, where around 80 per cent of participants are women. The postures were designed by men, for men's bodies, muscles and strength, and were practised from early childhood. When yoga was brought to the West, it was recognised by the early Indian teachers that our culture had no established programs of meditation or mind control. The ashtanga system with its focus on stillness, breathing and meditation was recognised as being initially very difficult for Westerners to grasp with our untrained minds. In a highly physical culture, the asana aspect was the obvious one to teach, and so it became the symbol of yoga. Many Western practitioners saw the benefits of the asana practice and continued to pursue the wisdom of yoga through its other limbs. The perceived cultural barriers of the Sutras, however, mean that yoga as a physical practice dominates, along with the secular hybridised versions that have evolved in gyms and elsewhere.

Most of us in the West would have met yoga through the postures, and probably had many teachers who never made the bigger spiritual connection with the other parts of the Sutras in which the asanas are found. While I have concentrated so far on hammering home the benefits of the mind and managing its unruly ways, the body as the sensory home of the mind is an essential element in your practice and good hustle. Much like there is a tendency to see yoga as an asana practice, there is also a strong tendency in Western cultures to view the body as who we are and strongly identify the physical as the 'real' self.

This makes a lot of sense in a culture where we are not steeped in a tradition of reincarnation that views the body as merely a convenient vehicle for this turn around in our human incarnation. Understanding the body as a solid and permanent feature of our identities strongly roots our attachment to the physical and aesthetic aspects of who we are as essential and unchanging. You can see in relation to attachment and consequent suffering where the problems begin using this mindset. Our bodies become our business cards; judgement, criticism and a relentless, punishing life of trying to conform ensue. At each interaction with other bodies we compare and contrast, continually holding ourselves separate from everyone else. We identify in our differences, and in our lack.

Our approach to our bodies and their differences is particularly human in our classifications and judgements. We would never walk into a forest and look across the trees and say, 'That one is too tall, that one too short, that one has too much bark and not enough leaves up top'.

We simply accept and delight in the vast diversity that nature offers in all her plants and beings. Your body is a similar offering. It is your instrument of movement, mind and action, nothing more. You need to keep it in the shape and form it needs to work properly over a lifetime, without overindulgence or abandonment. Just regular scheduled maintenance. And you need to love each of the other bodies as you walk through the forest of our worlds.

Asana has a valuable place in our yogic and good hustle practice, and can definitely be the salve that begins to soften and heal our approach to ourselves. As a tool for healing and therapy, the benefits of a yoga practice have been proven comprehensively. Interestingly, one of the reasons asana works in the process of healing both physically and emotionally is that it gets us out of our heads and into a physical practice. The concentration required to harmonise the breath and the body (in theory) leave little room for distractions by the mind. This is yet another method of neural pathway rebuilding. By integrating the body and the breath in a practice that leaves participants feeling a sense of peace and union, the body can take on the role of healer and nurturer. B.K.S. Iyengar says, 'Health begins with firmness in the body, deepens to emotional stability, then leads to intellectual clarity, wisdom and finally the unveiling of the soul.'

The daily asana session on the mat has a lot to offer us as entrepreneurs, especially in the early stages. The practice of asana is essential for us to be strong and flexible. In the spirit of a life devoted to, and in service for, others, the desire to remain fit and healthy is not about wanting to live forever for the sake of youth and beauty. It is instead entirely about utilising the longevity of our bodily vehicles to help us serve and gather enough integrated experiential wisdom to do so. We are watching in real time the inhabitants of the Western world being felled by chronic diseases. These epidemics are driven through lifestyles of over-attachment to sense objects, a lack of movement and a lack of preparation for our bodies to get as old as they are now able to do in the modern world. Yoga asana builds strength and flexibility to counter the aging of our muscles and tendons. This alone is a worthy reason for everyone to adopt a daily practice, even just as training to be able to bend over and pick their socks up off the floor in their eighties.

Time spent on the mat is not peripheral to our minds. As our bodies work through the combinations of muscle stretching and breath work we are engaged in a quest for the integration of our most precious tools. Through yoga asana practice, especially in the early years when our bodies are not the graceful origami of veteran yogis and are more like piles of pick-up sticks wobbling around, yoga challenges our perceived barriers. As I have mentioned before, we are so limited in what we believe is possible. Without experience, we are bound to only conceive what we know, and the rest seems as distant and intangible as clouds. When we see certain postures in yoga, or attempt them, we are certain that we will never be able to attain the shape our body is required to get into. Until one day we realise that our muscles are longer, our balance solid, our reach further, and we are suddenly there, at the place that once seemed impossible. A new frontier is formed, and a new horizon appears, then our questing continues to the next distant posture.

Asana is the physical expression of how we master ourselves. Our mind is kind of slippery—we think we have it, then realise that our hands are empty and it is again out of our grasp. It is a daily challenge that, unlike climbing Mount Everest, we can do with minimal risk, minimal resources and maximum benefit. Much like the realisations that result from the niyama practices of austerity, asana proves that over time we can do the things we believed were impossible.

Conquering these limiting self-beliefs is fundamental to being able to bring your good hustle from being a faraway idea to reality. When you take the time every day to grow yourself, you are giving yourself physical strength and discipline, both of which are needed to go the distance in your transition from life as a sense pleasure slave, chained to the bars of desire, to a detached and happy being at one with everything. Sequencing of asana postures requires us to move our bodies and minds from place to place without clinging to a posture that we might like because it feels good. Each asana is impermanent. In yoga asana, as we are subtly changing our minds to accept the expansion of our boundaries, so too are we inculcating agility and acceptance of the continual rapid change in our lives. Some of which we have control over, some of which we don't.

Agility is the key to survival in those first tentative steps into your good hustle venture, whether working in your own start-up, or as an intrapreneur for another enterprise. There will be many conditions that determine in the moment how you respond to an asana. You might be feeling stiff, or tired, or a little twingy, or not quite warmed up. All of those factors will determine how you enter and exit a pose. How your mind is chattering away will also determine whether you feel long and strong, or weak and unwilling, changing the shape of the expression of your asana. As you enter the market with your big, purposeful dream made real, subtle micro and macro determinants will change the way each day and each goal plays out. Your customers will ask for certain things, your suppliers may change an order, or a delivery, or suddenly cease to exist. You might find one product sells, where another is ignored or rejected by your customers. You might just find your server goes down on the day you had your big webinar scheduled, or a virus wipes out your database—you get the picture.

None of these things are ultimately good or bad, they are simply what is and what needs to be dealt with to move your day, your business and your project along. They will all take you to a new frontier, and some of them will seem like a gift, others make you want to run for the doona and settle in. What asana practice will translate from the mat to the laptop or shopfront is that all of these situations will flow, and your reaction to them will change from day to day. How you feel about the ever-changing moment is irrelevant. Your reaction determines whether or not you get the job done efficiently. How you feel about one posture or another is similarly irrelevant, you have to move your body into the pose and out of it, no matter how you feel about it. How you feel about your body is similarly irrelevant; tall or short, fat or slim, freckled or wrinkly, it is what it is today, and tomorrow it will be subtly different. Overwhelmingly, however, a yoga asana practice is essential for keeping the vehicle of your body on the road that ultimately leads to the experience of the divine.

4. Pranayama

This fourth stage of the ashtanga process consists of techniques designed to gain control over breathing while recognising the connection between the breath, the mind and the emotions. Pranayama translates as life-force expansion, and yogis believe, with a credible body of evidence, that it not only rejuvenates the body but extends life. 'Prana' is life force and energy, often achieved through breathing practices. 'Ayama' is a stretching, a regulation, a control, thus pranayama is an expansion of our life force and a stretching of our capacity through breath control. Not a stretch to see why it is such an integral and important part of a yoga practice. Pranayama in an asana routine can be undertaken at the commencement and conclusion of a yoga practice as well as within the postures, or used as a stand-alone breathing practice at any time.

The first four stages of Patanjali's ashtanga yoga concentrate on understanding our personalities, gaining skill in controlling the body, and developing an awareness of ourselves. The body, while not separate from the mind, is a gross tool of the sense organs and a significant distraction from the journey towards a higher state of consciousness if not under strict control. Patanjali noted that the breath is a vehicle for achieving an awareness of our consciousness. We need to learn to slowly and systematically measure and manipulate its distribution. Understanding the vital role breath plays in stilling the mind and the body, it is also important to remember that breath is not under our control. In this light, we can look at our relationship with it in terms of pranayama as one of collaboration and negotiation—also key skills to master for our good hustle practice. Breath will come in and out. The amount of actual attention you have paid to breathing since your birth is miniscule.

Breath doesn't need you as the doer, and this in itself is invaluable wisdom to remember. All of the time your mind has spent applying itself to planning control of and attachment to the things that you believe are the most essential to your survival (reputation, good Instagram selfies, consuming rainbow layer cakes) is time you haven't spent on your breath. All the drama, the days when life seemed like it was literally going to end because of some heartbreak, criticism, disappointment or disaster, you just kept on breathing, and living.

Breath as the most critical element to your life is seemingly a free agent, blissfully decoupled from your mind and its distractions, able to single-pointedly get on with delivering essential services day and night. There is much we can learn from our breath, and perhaps the best lesson is humility. Our mind needs to be reminded that it can pretend to be the boss all it likes, but everything we actually need is within, patiently performing and waiting to be noticed. If you are a yoga teacher or student, you will have heard this phrase many times: come back to the breath. The breath is the constant that we orient our practice around, it is the central golden cord of releasing distraction and returning to stillness and awareness. Breath similarly anchors meditation practices. We follow its path in and out of our nostrils with wonder each time we return, as if seeing the miracle of our breathing for the first time. The gratitude and eager embrace of breath as something to anchor us to settle our minds is soon lost again as the rainclouds of thought return, and the process of loss and gaining of consciousness continues.

When we talk about training our breath in yoga, we are really training our bodies to recognise that breath is there and available to us. We can slow it down, deepen it, extract healing powers from it, and regulate the reaction of our bodies and minds. The breath within those actions doesn't fundamentally change. We change around it. Pranayama teaches us the fundamental requirement as entrepreneurs to trust and surrender to that we don't control. These layer together when we make breath a conscious and central part of our practice in a loop of remembrance and surrender. It is the physical and lived experience of that wisdom. What we need to grasp is that despite what happens around it, breath just keeps going. It's not attached to anything. This is how we need to model ourselves as we move down the path of ideation into the set-up of our new businesses.

We need to keep moving in a regular rhythm, paying attention without attachment, and making decisions based on simply moving the concept forward, breath by breath.

If pranayama is the extension of our vital life-force energy through breathing practice, and we are summoning this life force to help us with the monumental task required to shift our mindsets, it stands to reason that we are going to need to harness and cultivate quantities of energy. We need to generate prana and we need to consciously work with our asana and pranayama practice to do so. As we increase strength, fortitude and resilience in the body, so too the breath as the vehicle of our consciousness and awareness needs to be cultivated.

If you aren't a current practitioner of pranayama, start today. Start right now. Just sit, book or Kindle in hand or headphones on, and focus on the breath. Connect to the idea that nothing happens without it, and it happens with nothing originating from your conscious thinking mind. Simply deepening the quality of your inhalations is going to be a boon for your health. You can start with a couple of minutes a day—include it in your yoga asana practice, or on waking and retiring, but the key part is to make it a conscious practice and link that neural pathway to unlocking your own inner intelligence. Pranayama is not just breathing—be mindful of the subtle difference. It is the harnessing and stoking of energy, building the furnace to fuel your inner workings to new heights. What else might be sitting silently inside you, working on autopilot, waiting for a chance to be uncovered as you quieten the mind? This is an actual process, rather than an intellectual one.

It starts with using pranayama as a tool to calm the mind, still our bodies and energise ourselves. It may feel a little strange at first, as though you are having a conversation with yourself, but persist. The shift will come when you trust yourself, and realise that you have the answers, if you choose to listen.

These days I'm a great consulter of my inner wisdom or however you want to characterise this innate voice. I quiet down and engage my breath, and focus my mind on my interior world, which will of course look, feel and be perceived differently for everyone. When I first started this practice of inner consultation, I'd ask myself a question, and an answer would snap back at me. I was convinced I was just talking to myself; after all, that voice sounded the same as the one that was the critical inner monologue that had been my life companion. I came to realise that while the voice sounded the same, it was definitely not me. It was the quality of the response that was different. There wasn't a sense of outcomes being good or bad—there was simply advice being given. I didn't have to be anything or anyone different; I was being given the advice unconditionally, without prejudice. I could choose to use or ignore it, and I knew that the outcome would be furthering me whatever I chose. But I also knew that I got an honest answer; so much so that now, if I suspect I won't like what I'm going to hear, I might delay the asking.

This inner wisdom is not something special to me. It's not something you have to take a course on, or do ten different levels of initiation at escalating costs to enjoy, despite what you may see advertised. Every one of us has access, all the time, but we need to prepare the ground to hear. With your inner voice, just ask the question that you want answers to in a simple and straightforward way, and wait for the answer. As I said, it might take you a little while to learn to recognise your own divinity at work. But persevere.

As you develop ideas for your good hustle endeavours, link the practice of pranayama to sessions where you are working on ideation and creativity. As you would engage your core to sustain a yoga pose, engage your breath to sustain your mental acuity. When you hit a big decision, or a stressful moment, engage your breath to bring everything back to an even keel. Take the energy that might be stuck in your chest or throat and redistribute it around your whole body and return your sympathetic nervous system to its regular program. While the breath doesn't need your control, you can certainly collaborate with it when you body gets out of kilter through external stresses and shocks. When your concentration is lacking through tiredness (those new austerity measures of getting up early can take some adjustment) you can binge on pranayama, not chocolate, to re-energise your afternoon or evening and continue getting the work done for your good hustle project. Our breath is a potent teacher of many lessons and a constant force to be used on our journey inwards. Pranayama is a critically important practice and one that deserves attention and integration into our daily lives.

5. Pratyahara

Pratyahara is the continuation of turning inwards and starting to address the world outside of our constant sensory stimulus. This stage is always represented to me in the part of every yoga class where vigorous action slows, eyes are closed, and you are taken out of your physical exertions and into the gentle passage to savasana. It is no accident that even within the structure of a yoga class, we are replicating a microcosm of the yamas and niyamas in every posture and breath. The practice of pratyahara provides us with an opportunity to step back into the role of observer or witness: to impartially and compassionately look at ourselves and really see who we are. In doing so, we can take the opportunity to catalogue the parts of ourselves that serve us, and the parts that don't, without contributing to our own suffering with self-criticism and harsh words.

Silence, stillness and contemplation are not a big part of Western culture. We like noise and distractions. Consequently our minds have become the equivalent of having the TV blaring on a shopping channel 24/7. We are so attached to external stimulus, to things and what we see as the permanent tangibles of life that define our experience of being, that the idea of turning in (or away from the outside) is one that is often hard to grasp. Like letting go, it is a phrase that is maddeningly free of detailed instructions. The sense is that we can simply release and move on, but as everyone knows, this is far easier said than done.

The work of pratyahara doesn't mean that you can't be working on your good hustle plan at the same time. All of this can be travelling in parallel, but the awakening of the dharma is the priority at the outset. The only way to get there is to turn in, and deal with what has been stopping you. Pratyahara is the limb when you are really committing to do the deep work, armed with the emerging dialogue with your own innate wisdom. This is the practice that leads to your divinity, and your dharma. The sirens of your attachments continue to call throughout each limb; this is the fundamental nature of distraction.

So how, why and when do we turn in? Pranayama, our breathing practice, is the precursor to pratyahara, both in the sequence of the eight limbs and in the action of turning focus to the breath. We bring the prana inside to build consciousness and energise our entire bodies. It is here we are already renouncing the outside world for the inky mystery of our internal realms. The breath straddles the cusp of our extroverted body, and our introverted inner world. This is where we find the mind, and the process of pratyahara takes us from a place of looking and seeing in our externally focused view, to listening to our inner voice, our inner wisdoms. On the inside, the ego seems to have fewer places to grip. Without the familiar visual cues of the body and world to give us place and context, turning in gives us little to grasp, decoupling our familiar dualities and creating space for new ways of thinking and being. This is how we can work on change in ourselves. Switching down the lights and gently pushing ourselves into finding new ways of getting around, wearing new tracks in our minds. Once the disorientation of being effectively blindfolded against our primary senses occurs, there begins the sensation of freedom and potential, where our awareness is released into infinite space. This is the moment in meditation that I am most attached to, when I leave the wriggling and adjusting and mental cataloguing, and have the first sensation of emptiness and dropping down within. For those tiny moments it feels like freefall as the outer world is nullified and time takes on a new dimension.

It is developing the discipline of asana and moving to a breathing practice that prepares us for the new senses and sensations of pratyahara. With our external senses we engage in an acquisition process—we see things, we judge them, we identify them, we relate them to us and attach labels like good or bad, want or don't want, all the usual dualities that keep us busy, separate and miserable. Pratyahara takes that sense shopping away, and rather than the public cavalcade of desire, offers us up our internal catalogue, which is infinitely less desirable. The discipline is to stay focused, stay present, simply observing as the raw and uncensored explosion of your mind pours forth. Yes, it is a visceral and often confronting experience. My attachment to the opening moments of entering the space of internal contemplation is no doubt a response to the battle that is quick to follow of taming and controlling my thoughts. Without all of the sense pleasures to keep me distracted, in pratyahara I'm confronted by the spectre of my mental torments and temptations.

If I want to focus on the breath, I can be sure that my mind wants me to focus on the itching on my face, the pins and needles in my foot, the delicious meal I yearn for, a deeply shameful thought I had relegated to the back of my mind, the piercing hurt of betrayal or rejection that brings instant pain to my being. These are the mind battles that I and so many people experience every time we sit down and turn within. It's no wonder that despite the known benefits of meditation, many of us choose to not run this gauntlet in the practice of taming our unruly minds.

The antidote to the cacophony of internal chatter in silent meditation is what amounts to a process of tag and release. Non-attachment lies here; it is where the practice of letting go and detaching from emotion and reaction begins. A thought arises, we note it, superficially examine its root cause and relation to previous thoughts, and then release it. Whatever it is, tag and release. Don't hold on, deep dive, reiterate and resolve; simply note that a thought has come, you recognise it, and now it can go.

With practice in the practice, there is a pattern to what appears regularly in our thoughts, and with familiarity the process becomes quicker. The temptation to explore, to follow our thoughts down the rabbit holes of our mind, and to indulge the fictional narratives that accompany our version of life, is a constant struggle. The torment and busyness definitely lessens as we train ourselves to keep dismissing and coming back. But there is often a sense of things getting worse, and a feeling that you will never get past the whirling dervishes of your mind. You will.

When and where in our good hustle practice do we engage the process of pratyahara? The limb of pranayama reminded us of the truth about our control over essential services—or not. We sought inner wisdom through the non-conscious nature of breathing. As we release the doing, in pratyahara we dive into the being. Here we see the mud being stirred up by our minds as we endeavour to settle and eventually see clarity in the water of our thoughts. By withdrawing the senses and seriously attending to managing your mind, you are polishing the diamond of your self. In this action you are enabling the inner vision of who you are, and what is most going to serve you. For all the marketing hype around the idea of doing what you love meaning never working a day in your life, this needs to be balanced with the reality of the internal work that has to be done every day. It doesn't mean that you won't love doing it. It's an essential part of the path to your own growth and freedom from suffering. But this is, as frequently reiterated, a lifetime commitment, with much of it spent in an inward-facing position.

Pratyahara teaches us the skills of tagging and releasing our thoughts without attachment. While this is applied to our inner work, it can also be applied to our outer work. The distractions that call us away from the mundane but necessary tasks of planning and researching our new ventures, budgeting, strategising and doing the things we find hard and distasteful, are a constant in life. We can translate the discipline from our practice of pratyahara of acknowledging the call to turn our attention elsewhere, and the root that drives it, and return to our work, knowing that our concentration is required.

6. Dharana

Each stage of the eight limbs can be plucked out and used individually, but collectively, they lead to union in lock step. The practice of pratyahara creates the setting for dharana, or concentration. Having removed outside distractions by withdrawing the senses, we can continue to deal with the far more intrusive and overwhelming distractions of the mind itself.

In the practice of dharana, we learn to slow down the thinking process by concentrating. Using the role of the observer, dismissing thoughts after we have tagged and released them is the first part of the procedure to still our minds. This isn't so much concentration, although it does require a sustained effort. Once the chatter, clatter, snapping and sniping is managed, the concentration part of meditation can test the efficacy of our new mind muscles to hold the errant thoughts at bay. This can be done using classic techniques of meditation when the puppy or monkey mind is tethered to the post of a single mental object. Sometimes a tethered puppy will sit quietly awaiting its owner's return or command. Other times, it will pull and squirm and whine until acknowledged and given its way. The tethering of the puppy mind is a similarly unpredictable excursion. Find a tether point that is somewhat comfortable or compelling for you to visualise, that you can commit your time to. This can be anything you can imagine, but commonly people choose a specific place in the body such as the third eye or above the navel or a chakra. It can be an image of a deity or guru, a candle flame, the entry and exit point of the breath, or silent repetition of a sound such as *aum* or *ram*.

Initially the introduction of a point of concentration is in itself a distraction, and for at least a couple of seconds, it seems possible to focus on a single point, without it being shredded and scattered to the four corners of the mind. All too swiftly you realise that while you started out watching the flame, that quickly morphed into self-congratulation about your powers of meditation. From there you snuck into a maze of mildly related concepts, and the flame of single-pointed concentration was well and truly snuffed out. Like the discipline of pratyahara, the only course is to come back to the flame or your point of tether over and over and over again. During this repetition you begin to realise that the point of concentration is not in holding the image, it is in the shortness of time between realising you have let go and coming back and starting over. There is a saying that dharana can't be taught, only caught. In knowing that, you can practise catching as well as concentrating.

I mentioned earlier opportun-itis being one of the pitfalls of the ideation stage of creating your good hustle, where there are so many opportunities that you want to grab that you end up not being able to execute any of them. I'm sure you've picked up right away the reason that the limb of dharana in yoga is necessary. Concentrating on one thing is a skill that is being systematically dismantled in our culture. When the term multi-tasking entered the lexicon, it became a desirable skill, one that indicated the capacity for hyper-productivity and superior juggling of priorities. It's a must-have on your CV, and is seen as particularly useful for women, who are masterful at multi-tasking in their poly roles managing the household, caring for aging parents, raising children and completing study. Maintaining a career is now seamlessly integrated, with the other full-time work assumed. Our attention is trained to be on many things at once, and this has been compounded by the 'always on' state of our mobile devices. No longer do we simply watch TV. We also have conversations, eat dinner, engage on multiple social media channels and respond to email simultaneously. We're taking in vast quantities of information and trying to process it all in some meaningful way.

It's little wonder that anxiety is so widespread. It is stressful and exhausting to maintain that level of engagement over many hours, days and weeks. This gives us a clue as to why, when asked to let go and still the mind, it seems like a herculean task. This is the backdrop against which we need to ask how Patanjali would have advised his contemporary yogis to reach for their nirvana.

If our intention in knowing our own minds is a search for the root cause of our suffering, this is an easy undertaking. Too much communication is the symptom and an underlying anxiety of not being enough is the root of the pain. The simple solution is to reject the assertion that we need to be simultaneously connected and always available. Refuse to participate. Set your own agenda and boundaries for access that is acceptable to your pace and needs. It's that easy. Most of us haven't actually tested the hypothesis to see if the world ends when we don't have a device at our fingertips. In Buddhism, there is a set of precepts where one of the explicit undertakings is renouncing being human. It sounds overly dramatic and final but the breakdown of the idea is that as humans we are all hopelessly devoted to sense objects (or the eight worldly dharmas, which will be covered a little later), and because of that we are, from birth, in a state of suffering. The recommendation from one of the enlightened beings of Buddhism is that to break with the root of samsara, we have to break with our humanness. For you and me in our lives in transition to being good hustlers, it means that we are accepting that, gradually, as we get further into our spiritual practices and our search for self, the sense pleasures and material attachments that our fellow humans are oriented to are no longer our motivations. We don't want to go to the pub, or gossip and snipe about others, or binge on Netflix series, or play Minecraft for twelve hours, or fixate on food, booze, pills and their consumption. In making these choices, we remove our 'humanness' as we remove our attachments to the primary causes of suffering. It is a big and interesting concept, which also loops us back to the heart of the idea of impermanence. If we aren't what we know to be the label of human, what and who are we? The answer is, it doesn't really matter, if what we are is compassionate and loving.

Disciplining ourselves to undertake one single-pointed task at a time is another way of retraining that part of us that has forgotten what concentration feels like. I regularly experience this while I am doing something like writing, or trying to deliver a project to deadline. While deep in thought, suddenly, as if compelled by outside forces, I will find myself reaching for my phone to look at email or social media. It's infuriating, as by the time I realise what is happening, I've lost my flow and have to then capture my concentration again and return to the sentence. Nothing needs me in any instant, but I need the comfort of my own distractions.

You need to return to the nostalgic ways of concentration; we all do. I've noticed over the years that one of the constant traits of entrepreneurs is the capacity for an inherent, almost unconscious adoption of similar practices that are used in yogic disciplines. Entrepreneurs are able to see and hold a single point of focus no matter what distractions and hardships come across their path. They may well flow around them, or be agile in their approach to achieving their goal, but even though the method may change, they are able to successfully hold their focus.

Cultivating concentration in the pursuit of your good hustle doesn't have to be a practice just directed at turning off your devices to complete a piece of work. It is also a social and interactive action that can and should be used in interactions with each other. I like to consciously engage dharana when talking to someone, giving them my single-pointed attention, rather than listening with one ear, checking texts and thinking about my next meeting or some other problem. By maintaining a sensory focus on actively listening to and looking at them, taking in the full experience of being in the moment with that person, the richness of information gathered is exquisite, and the exchange is loving and meaningful.

Service to others sits here. It is a service to people when we truly connect and listen, and give them our full attention; when we see and hear them in their completeness, and reflect back to them through our actions that they are worthy of our time and attention. This is an act of devotion. It can and should also be an act of unconditional love, as there need be no expectation of anything other than that moment of connection.

In a brand and customer sense, bringing this individualised concentration to interactions is a display of pure authenticity, that buzz word that symbolises the cut-through which all businesses are looking for. It doesn't come from slick marketing and strategising. In a service-oriented enterprise it comes from genuinely realising that customers don't simply exist for a transactional exchange to build your revenue. They exist as individuals, and humans, and are the sentient beings that your heart longs to integrate with. When we undergo the practice of creating a persona of our customer for marketing purposes, we are doing far more than homogenising a template of our ideal target for sales. That is an entirely conditional viewpoint that only looks to what benefits you can get, rather than what you can give. When working on understanding who your ideal customer is, undertake the exercise of creating a persona to design a clearly defined customer. This person is the one to whom you can offer the most service, and deliver your promise of unconditional love and compassion. This is a significant part of the good hustle mindset.

7. Dhyana

Meditation or contemplation, the seventh stage of ashtanga, is the uninterrupted flow of concentration. Although mindful concentration and meditation seem to be practically identical, there are infinite differences. Where dharana practises one-pointed attention, dhyana is the ultimate state of being acutely aware but renouncing focus. The mind has been quieted by the preceding activities and disciplines learned through the other limbs. In the stillness you have created, the production of thoughts is reduced to a minimum (theoretically at least). Dhyana is where all the practice has been leading. Learning the ability to slow it all down and look within enables the work on awareness and self to be integrated. We've covered much of the territory that leads us here as we worked through Patanjali's recipe for becoming yogi. Now we are at the destination of dhyana, the practice itself is like a whole new beginning, bringing a new set of learnings.

As one of the seminal texts on yoga as a system of living, the Bhagavad Gita is integral to good hustle practices. Krishna's advice in the Gita on meditation is a perfect companion to where we have landed. In the Gita, Krishna makes a passionate defence of the benefits of meditation. Our other protagonist, Arjuna, is in a state of emotional paralysis over starting the battle of Kurukshetra. He is slumped in the bottom of his chariot, weapons down, unable to motivate himself to get up and begin fighting. Arjuna as a fierce warrior, at this point, is displaying character traits more akin to those of a whiny child, as he pouts and sulks in answer to Krishna's increasingly firm entreaties to bring some mindful action into the moment.

This is a place all of us have been to. I encounter it regularly when the alarm goes off to get up for meditation; or to go to a yoga class; or to start a piece of work or edit a manuscript. It's a place where you just can't take the next step. You know you must, you know that when you do it will be good for you, you'll enjoy it. And yet there you are slumped at the bottom of your own chariot; your mind filling you up with thoughts of all the other things you could do, and all the reasons to stay exactly where you are.

Krishna throughout the Gita comes back again and again to meditation as the foundation of any imminent action. The Gita works as a text for those of us about to embark on making their dharma their life, as it is a reminder that while following that path is hard, it is far harder to do nothing and live a life empty of true purpose. Arjuna speaks for all of us when he counters Krishna's prescription for meditation by pointing out that meditation is hard, likening controlling the mind to controlling the wind. And Krishna's response?

Just keep practising.

Krishna is ardent about the practice of meditation as the key tool to reveal our true self and its nature. He gives

Arjuna explicit instructions on what to do: how to sit, how to breathe, the stages to work through. He teaches him yoga for life right there on the edge of the battlefield. Krishna says that the practice of meditation is the solution to us getting back our innate wisdom, the knowledge of who we are and what we are here to do. As long as we don't know who we are, or what to do, we remain actors, playing out roles that only ever reach a peripheral layer of our being. Sometimes we get so good at playing the role we stepped into that we never take off the mask and get typecast, unable to ever struggle out of our costumes and be ourselves. It takes courage to step out of being human and commit to searching for who we are, and a way to live in our truth.

Arjuna's feeling of paralysis is a common condition when you come across that one business idea that you know is going to be your ticket to dharma. There is an accompanying sensation of vastness mingled with sheer terror—this is what you see when the veil is removed, and for one clear moment you connect and are shown what life can be like. In the Gita, Arjuna asks Krishna to show him who he is—referring to his godly persona rather than his charioteer, childhood buddy image. Throughout the story Arjuna has only encountered Krishna in his human form, and while he knows he is possessed of godly powers, he wants the proof of Krishna's divinity.

When Krishna obliges by revealing his immortal self (reportedly an endless array of Krishna's many bodies, forms, powers and action all at once), Arjuna is completely overwhelmed. Krishna has blindsided him, and he struggles to recalibrate the idea of the Krishna he knows, and the infinite source of wonder that he just saw, begging Krishna to immediately return to his original flavour.

This is how we find ourselves paralysed and overwhelmed when we have the experience of seeing our own potential and our own divinity when we connect to our greater selves. Part of the paralysis lies in the simplicity of the solution, as both Krishna and Patanjali lay out in their own way: to follow your dharma, turn in, connect with your self, relinquish the 'I' for the selfless service to the greater humanity, meditate, and renounce attachment to results and objects through simply providing service. It is a straight-up prescription for the path of yoga, and both proponents guarantee the results are a life of meaning and joy. But as we know from understanding what is involved in the previous steps, it is difficult to relinquish the habits and patterns we have picked up over our lives, and in the collective culture we are born into. It's hard to stop being human, after all.

You can liken this process of letting go, and the difficulty of releasing your grip, to the imaginal cells of a caterpillar undergoing its metamorphosis to a butterfly. The caterpillar has within it the cells of change for its cyclical evolution. When the process begins, the caterpillar body fights the cells that appear to bring about the change, seeing them as an enemy of its immune system. As the internal battle rages between caterpillar cells and butterfly cells, eventually the balance shifts, and the number of butterfly cells outweighs those caterpillar cells that are holding on to the old form and old ways of being. Once this balance is tipped, the new cells can do their work, bringing forth the butterfly. We are all caterpillars, feeling the emergence of the innate understanding in us that change is necessary for us to evolve. But our imaginal cells fight it, and cling to the things that have previously served us, the behaviours and feelings that we know, even if only on a conscious level, aren't serving us.

The metaphor of Arjuna's battle is apt, as making change in our life, finding our good hustle, often feels like a battle. It's confusing and exhausting, and all we want is for it to be over and peace to reign. This is where the story of the Gita is so familiar and relatable. Arjuna is at the point of collapse, in a painful identity crisis. He knows the war of Kurukshetra is necessary and to a degree inevitable, and that there is no quick and easy way to get it over with, as all civil negotiations have failed. The battle is going to change the face of civilisation. Arjuna is unable to see beyond the now to the greater benefits he will experience once the fighting is over. He is desperately looking for ways to maintain the status quo, to keep everyone happy, while knowing that this solution will result in no one being happy. When we make change in ourselves, especially when these changes begin to reveal the truth of our own inner butterflies, there is a ripple effect without and within. Resistance will come from your peers, your colleagues, your family and loved ones.

We are all sleeping caterpillar cells, and the awakening butterfly of one of us challenges the rest to look at their own lives and take inventory of their sense of fulfilment and purpose. You will undoubtedly be challenged both gently and critically when you start to reveal that you aspire to renounce your attachments and seek a life of dharma.

These reactions will happen, I guarantee it, when you first broach the idea of, say, leaving your job to pursue your good hustle ideas. The prevailing idea in society seems to be that it is better to be unhappy and unfulfilled than seek to step outside of the suffering and try. Treasure the humans who instantly get where you are coming from and encourage you. Keep them in your inner circle and invite them to be part of your process of growth.

It's best to avoid evangelising and trying to convince others to follow once you have leapt into your good hustle zone, as each of us has to work through the eight steps at our own pace. We have to have collapsed in our chariots and thrown our hands in the air wondering if this is all there is, surrendering to our version of Krishna for answers to our despair. And of course the answers come, and they come from within, and they come through preparing ourselves to hear the gentle whisper of our heart through reaching the stage of dhyana.

The strength and stamina it takes to reach this state of stillness are quite impressive—think of a dam wall holding up a crashing, thundering expanse of water. And it certainly feels to the meditator that there are too many holes and not enough fingers. But remember this patience and observance are in themselves part of the process. There is growth and benefit at every stage of our progress and in the spirit of the seeker; reaching the end is not the goal, it is the experience of living the practice that helps us reach the end and our goal: samadhi.

8. Samadhi

Patanjali describes this eighth and final stage of ashtanga, samadhi, as a state of ecstasy. At this stage, the yogi merges with their point of focus and transcends the self altogether. A profound connection to the divine is realised and there is an interconnectedness with all living things. Read this not as a lofty and unachievable religious or spiritual goal. If we return to our earlier discussion of how we individually define the divine, this merging is with that divinity that delivers us peace, contentment and happiness. Not just for ourselves, but through knowing that this is a state bestowed on all things. The state of enlightenment isn't like falling through a rabbit hole into the inky nothingness of thoughtless ecstasy—samadhi is a state of action and equanimity. This is the goal for your good hustle. It is a thoroughly ambitious undertaking, delivering you to a place far greater than the individual 'I', as you provide service to the world and gain samadhi as a result. As Krishna tells Arjuna in the Gita, there is a certain kind of action that leads to freedom and fulfilment. Krishna and the Gita are full of kernels of wisdom for the dharma seeker that reinforce the peril of stasis. Reiterating the call to arms for those of us who have begun to wake up and feel the creeping sense of dissatisfaction with the things (and they are things) that we used to think brought happiness. Denying your yearning for something more meaningful is in itself an action, and as we have discussed, karma is accrued with all actions. If action is unavoidable, we might as well make sure that it is action that points us in the direction of our own divinity.

The trick of the light is that divinity is, should, and can be, a very everyday event. It is in fact the everydayness of it that makes samadhi a worthwhile and achievable goal, and inextricably links it to good hustle. In trying to snap Arjuna out of his malaise, Krishna is continually reiterating that the pursuit of dharma *is* the way to divinity—and a portal to samadhi when done right. What is clear from Krishna's message in the Gita is that finding your dharma happens through taking action, and is one of the action steps not attached to the fruits of labour. This is what separates your good hustle: that the actions you are taking are not motivated by your own self-aggrandisement. Dedicating your business practice to something bigger than you decouples the way you approach work. No longer does it only exist for you and your limited worldview. It exists as an integral part of the world.

Gandhi is perhaps one of the greatest exponents of the shift in perspective when living a life dedicated to a good hustle and of what can be achieved. His dedication to not being human has made him an enduring icon of morality and ethics to all humanity. Gandhi's life was transformed when he first read the Gita. In his autobiography he details how up to that point his life had been somewhat of a litany of failure and shame—at least from the perspective of his family. Gandhi's identification with the fears and neurosis of Arjuna enabled him to take the advice of Krishna. Gandhi wholeheartedly surrendered himself to the process of finding out what his purpose was. He changed his diet, his friends and radically simplified his way of living. He took to daily meditation and mantra practice.

Gandhi, in his profession as a lawyer, had been just scraping by on his shallow legal knowledge. His final transformation came when he was working on a difficult and divisive case in South Africa between two families—spookily not unlike the Pandavas and Kauravas of the Gita. Although this had the potential to be very lucrative for Gandhi as a young lawyer, with years in litigation of the complex conflict spanning ahead of him, he could see the pain it was causing both sides and the damage that was being done. He made it his mission to convince the litigants to go to arbitration and drop the court case. When he successfully managed to negotiate a mutually acceptable compromise between them, it was the moment his own good hustle became clear: working to unite parties in conflict.

Knowledge became wisdom. Gandhi realised that when he was in union with his dharma, there was nothing that he couldn't attempt.

Gandhi wasn't a man blinded by faith or beguiled by religion without wisdom. In his desperate search for meaning in his life while living in England and studying, he had vigorously researched the seminal texts of all the world's major religions to try to discover something that gave him insight into finding peace and happiness. He concluded that all of the texts more or less prescribed the same thing, and no matter what culture and faith we are born into, we are all at heart looking within for the path to our true selves. For Gandhi the Gita was the book that gave a clear and simple step-by-step approach how to do so; a method that any seeker could adopt and use within their own belief system. Gandhi's commentary on the Gita, *The Bhagavad Gita According to Gandhi*, is a beautiful and straightforward analysis of the text. In the book he relates Krishna's advice to Arjuna to everyday situations, with the belief that the teachings should be accessible, understandable and actionable for everyone, from heads of state to street vendors, ensuring that enlightenment wasn't just a conceit for the elite.

The combination of action with the idea of a lack of attachment, as we have trained ourselves for in the previous eight limbs of the Sutras, is essential in your preparation for the creation of your good hustle. The single act of mastering non-attachment is in itself a form of samadhi. What better way to experience the absence of suffering than not being a slave to endless litanies of objects and emotions built on a foundation of your own destructive fictions.

This is freedom.

As Gandhi discovered, with surrender to the known unknown and selfless service as the motivator of all action, there is little that can't be achieved. As Krishna says in the Gita, 'Performing action without attachment, [wo] man shall attain the Supreme.' When the 'I' of the ego isn't attached to action, the limitations are removed. You don't attach your inner patterns of not being enough to what you are doing, creating a self-fulfilling prophecy of failure and shame. You merely get on and begin, knowing that you are being guided by your inner wisdom, which is now a clear, strong voice after the training of the Sutras.

The legacy that Gandhi left to the world as an exemplar of living a life in an entirely authentic and imperfect way has been expansive; the change he achieved was nothing short of miraculous. We can learn subtler lessons from Gandhi by studying the source of his courage and prescience that enabled him to undertake the breathtakingly subversive acts of nonviolence that freed his people from British rule. As part of his adherence to the teachings of the Gita, Gandhi relied entirely on his inner voice and moral compass. He used extended periods of concentration and meditation to guide his actions, and had no qualms in changing his direction in a dramatic and unexpected way if he felt he was being guided to do so. Such was his faith in surrender and following his dharma. By choosing his own access to understanding what the right path was, Gandhi wasn't swayed by opinion or tethered to what others thought.

Gandhi modelled agility and a reliance on his intuition, skills indubitably honed by his strict yoga and meditation practice. While in London he had practised the austerity of simplifying his life, ridding himself of unnecessary possessions, at the same time as he was working through cleaning his mind. In Gandhi's autobiography, *The Story of My Experiments with Truth*, he talks about the expansive freedom he felt, the less he had. It's a concept that is almost unimaginable to so many of us as we strive almost exclusively to acquire, or to pay for the things we have already acquired. His renunciation, however, was not about leaving the world and hanging in a cave or monastery. This is the legacy most useful to us as aspiring good hustle people, that we can have it all, we can do it all, by having none of it.

In the books and workshops run by motivational business coaches and successful entrepreneurs, so many familiar motivational catch phrases are trotted out. We need to have big, hairy, audacious goals (one of my most despised phrases); we need to be the change (coopted from one of Gandhi's own mantras); we need to fake it till we make it (see previous rant). There is a sense of striving and perpetual movement to reach the pinnacle of achievement that doesn't speak to the most important processes of silence: sitting, self-study, surrender and finally becoming one with ourselves, or with god, or however you conceive this practice of samadhi. One long-time yogi I spoke to was strongly of the opinion that we shouldn't even consider samadhi in our practice of becoming good hustlers; she felt it was not ever reachable. I counter this belief (which came from her context of spiritual practice) with the view that we *can* find our heavens on earth.

What Patanjali in the Sutras and Krishna in the Gita have described as the completion of the yogic path is, I believe, what, deep down, all of us aspire to: peace and contentment. A sense of purpose and meaning in our lives. This ultimate stage of yoga—enlightenment—can't be bought or possessed. It can only be experienced, and as such, it is the process of the practice, and is far more accessible than is realised. As you set out on your mission to find your good hustle, your strategy begins within. The first step is knowing who you are. You need to have a guiding motivation that you have surrendered to in love, and the courage of knowing that you can't fail when you are living in your dharma. The idea of failure is defunct when you aren't being measured against limited beliefs. You need to be confident that your nirvana, or samadhi or union with the divine, doesn't happen at the end of the rainbow. It *is* the rainbow and the reason for stepping out of what we experience as being human, and into the place of being *for* humanity instead. When you truly begin to break your attachment to objects and permanence, and realise the impermanent nature of everything, your loose grip on life will make everything simpler and you more content. If you can't control it, you don't have to worry about how you are going to, so you flow along and take opportunities as they present themselves, rather than as you create them. When you do create them, you do so with courage and without limitation, looking always to the single guiding principle that your motivation is to serve others with love, and contribute to the peace and happiness of all sentient beings.

This is the blueprint for good hustling. As Krishna broke it down in the Gita for Arjuna: find your dharma, look to it as you look within. Stay committed and disciplined, to get your mind in order until you have the clarity to see without doubt what is your calling. When you have seen that vision of your own capacity unlimited by your mortal flaws, do not let anything obscure your pursuit of delivering that goal to the world. 'Relinquish the fruits of your actions'; what Krishna intended by this was to give the outcomes and expectations away, and simply be nourished by the intention and the daily joys found in the present moment. Dedicate all of your actions to honouring your divinity, however you understand and experience that. This isn't an endgame, as the possibilities are such that you will experience moments of the essence of samadhi, moments of peace and contentment, that will push you along, and compel you to keep going until there is only keeping going, and what compels you is the sheer imperfect perfection of living in your dharma.

Pain and S(t)uffering

Throughout *The Good Hustle*, I've talked about attachment and material spirituality as things to be overcome, renounced and relinquished. It is why I am writing, and you are reading, this book, looking for a way to get back to you. Although it is woven throughout, I wanted to give this topic a dedicated space in the text, as it sits at the heart of suffering and the human condition.

I'm going out on a limb that if you are reading this, you are not living in a cave or a forest, at one with divinity, nibbling on roots and berries between meditation sessions. You are undoubtedly in the thick of the world, ticking each Kali Yuga day off the calendar. Until we really, deeply, truly get the problem with attachment, and make some inroads in our self-cherishing to kill it off at the root, attainment of good hustles, happy lives and peaceful hearts is elusive.

'What's Kali Yuga' I hear you say? I'm so glad you asked. You remember our friends Krishna and Arjuna at the edge of the battlefield, dealing with Arjuna's existential crisis? As we know, after a long and insightful talk by Krishna, Arjuna reconnects with his dharma, and saves the day upholding what is right by fighting for what is wrong—in his case the Pandavas' approach to grabbing land and people. Spoiler alert: Arjuna survives and morality along with him. Kali Yuga is, according to the Sanskrit scriptures, the age of the demon Kali. In the *Mahabharata* (the book from which the Bhagavad Gita is an excerpt) it is said that this age begins with the ending of the battle of Kurukshetra. The attributes of Kali Yuga were detailed as a spiritual dark age, where the emphasis on values shifted from faith, moral justice and the practice of the Hindu scriptures, to a time dominated by greed, violence and a general disregard for the types of conduct extolled in the Yoga Sutras.

There is in fact a spooky level of detail around the predictions of what would happen during the age of Kali Yuga in another Sanskrit classic, the *Srimad Bhagavatam*: 'Cities will be dominated by thieves, the Vedas will be contaminated by speculative interpretations of atheists [in other words, fake news], political leaders will virtually consume the citizens, and the so-called priests and intellectuals will be devotees of their bellies and genitals.' That feels awkwardly true right now.

Other predictions include the breakdown of inter-generational caring and support for parents; the rise of religious dogma to political power from 'non-spiritual' men; and an increase in the devastating impacts of snow, rain, fire and drought, putting pressures on populations for food and water security. Also predicted is the rise of wealth as a symbol of power; sex and physical attraction dominating love as a basis for relationships; and people developing a hatred for each other leading to the capacity to kill over minor differences. Yep. I think we've ticked all those boxes. Kali Yuga principally speaks to a loss of faith and of individuals caring for anything and anyone including nature, and the outcome this has for society and people. The age is predicted to last a long time (the end date is still hotly debated by Vedic mathematicians and astrologers, but it is estimated to be in around 423,000 years) and it doesn't end well. Human life gets shorter and shorter, and the inhabitants of once mighty civilisations are reduced to grubbing around for roots and berries to survive. But putting apocalyptic predictions to one side, Kali Yuga as described by Krishna in the Gita is a pretty accurate description of the state we find ourselves in now. The shift away from living with a collective desire for happiness, wellness and a lack of suffering; the absence of divinity that accepts and includes everyone (even and especially those who don't share your beliefs); and a solo and singular approach to living resulting in a sense of isolation and separateness, is a summation of the experience of life in the twenty-first century.

Whether or not you believe a document written 5000 years ago by a Hindu sage has relevance to where we find ourselves now, we can't argue with the generalised view that as countries accrue more wealth, and attain standards of living ever higher than previous generations, we appear sicker and unhappier than ever. So whether it is a function of Kali Yuga, or an excess of consumption combined with a high value placed on material wealth, it seems that the causal strand is a passionate attachment to things, leading to what Buddhists call suffering. I call it 'stuffering', as it is the acquisition and clinging to stuff in the belief that it is the root of happiness that is at the heart of most of our misery.

The Eight Worldly Dharmas

In Buddhism this stuff is known as the eight worldly dharmas or eight worldly concerns. These are kind of the opposite of the dharma we want to be cultivating; the eight worldly dharmas bind us to relationships with material objects. Where the Buddhadharma is the path to enlightenment, the eight worldly dharmas keep us trapped in samsara or suffering. These eight worldly dharmas (like everything) exist in the mind. The approach of Buddhism to the real and unreal, to reiterate, is that fundamentally we create things in our mind, and it is through our minds that we create the relationships and narratives about them. A book, for example, is made up of atoms, but when we look at a book, or hold a book, we think it is a solid piece of stuff. What we see and feel is a direct result of our experience of books. We classify and categorise the object and assign value—it's good or bad, and makes us nostalgic, reverent or excited—and see it and our relationship to it as permanent. Make sure you have your head around this as it is at the root of how attachment is understood, and how this leads to all things and our attachment to them being an illusion. If books aren't your thing (said no one ever), then do the same exercise with a pet: a living object made of protons, neutrons and electrons. You are unlikely to look at a dog and simply think this is an animal that is called a dog made of atoms. You would look at it and feel a rush of love, a desire to pat it, an attachment of value about its fur colour, texture and breed. Or alternately, if you had experienced negative interactions with dogs, you might experience fear, or revulsion, or anger, or even hunger depending on your cultural relationship to sources of protein.

None of these feelings change the reality of the makeup of that living object, but for you, that dog exists in your mind in a unique way that will not be experienced by anyone else. In both of these examples you experience attachment or aversion, cling to it, or desire to be free of the experience as soon as possible. In all things we 'know', we have created them in our minds, and understand them according to our personal experience. Attachment to what we have created and how we respond to it, in the Buddhist traditions, is samsara. It's suffering, and the only way to avoid the pain of stuffering is to renounce the world. Don't worry if your mind just exploded. Understanding impermanence can take lifetimes, and is a pretty serious philosophical road to go down. But like so many other big philosophical ideas we have bravely squared off against in *The Good Hustle*, the key is you know it is there, that these questions without answers exist, and that you can use them as a tool if and when it suits to help shape your own philosophies and beliefs.

The eight worldly dharmas are laid out in pairs and are as follows: the craving or attachment to something, and the craving to be free from craving for it; the craving for physical comfort and the aversion to discomfort; the craving for positive praise and the aversion to criticism; and the craving for a good reputation and the aversion to having your reputation trashed.

Attachment to Things/Craving to be Free from Craving

The first two are pretty common, and what we would generally recognise as attachment: craving for stuff and craving to be free from attachment to stuff. Along with possessions, I'd also add in food and other sensory consumables here. The craving for stuff is a serious problem for folks from the West to the East, from developing to very developed nations. This is the stuff of stuffering and we can't get enough of it. Literally. We know all the stages of stuff—wanting it, getting it, keeping it, disposing of it, sharing it, not sharing it, comparing it, being disappointed with it—and we know stuff doesn't make us happy. Even if we are adopting a sincere attitude of having a light footprint and divesting ourselves of stuff, there is the reverse suffering of being attached to not getting attached, and doing without. This includes the pride and judgement that attaches to being righteous about how good we are at saying no to stuff.

Which is simply another form of having an attachment. It's a tricky space to navigate, and it does sometimes feel impossible to get the balance right.

The point about attachment and the eight worldly dharmas, as I understand it, is not that we can't have the objects, it is the subtlety of both not attaching to having them *or* to not having them. As soon as we love them, or want them, or need them, or have pride about having them (or not having them), then we are captive to them and are attached. If we instead celebrate the comfort or pleasure they bring in the moment, but can sincerely release that desire instantly (not to go to a new attachment), then we are simply flowing with what is, in the moment. Lama Zopa Rinpoche reiterates this view. He says that wealth is not the problem, the problem is having desire for wealth. Friends are not the problem; attachment to our friends is. Objects become a problem for us because of the emotional mind of desire.

Craving Comfort/Aversion to Discomfort

The next pairing of the eight worldly dharmas comes with the same inherent dilemmas. Craving happiness and comfort, which is a strong signifier of success in our lives, is equalled in force with craving to be free from unhappiness and discomfort. There is also within these cravings another bridge of attachment, which is a fear of losing the comfort and happiness you have already attained. You're trapped coming or going. Happiness and its pursuit is the locus for so much suffering, and the problem lies not in any of the things of the external world, it lies within our mind. When we equate happiness with any of the eight worldly dharmas, which are what constitutes our Western understandings of happiness, not one of them is linked to our internal state of being, or our capacity for connection to others and our own divinity. The achievement of this state, gained by releasing our minds from illusions through yoga, meditation, living in dharma, and offering ourselves in love, is where happiness lies. This is not what we are told about happiness and comfort from our earliest arrival into the world.

We're referencing Abraham H. Maslow's hierarchy of needs to understand what the basic elements of survival and thrival are for humans. Maslow, a psychologist, released his heavily adopted theory of human self-actualisation in 1943, with his paper 'A Theory of Human Motivation'. In it, he created a pyramid that is a neat summation of the eight worldly dharmas: all of his prescriptions for happiness are provided by external sources. In this context, it is completely understandable how and why everything we do and see is predicated on happiness and comfort being given to us, and therefore, at constant risk of being taken away. It is all in our mindset and approach to the encounters we have with what we believe is happiness and comfort, and our reaction to it. Consider temperature. On a hot summer's day, we encounter a room that is cool. We were sweating in the heat, drowning in humidity, hot and bothered with the world and desperate to get some respite. The heat of the day and getting away from it were completely dominating our thoughts. We were caught in suffering. When we encounter an air-conditioned space, our day and feeling of happiness are transformed, it is blissful, cool, we calm down, our mood becomes light and joyful. Cool makes us happy. Heat makes us suffer. We want to avoid heat, and encounter cool. Then the opposite occurs. In winter, cool does not make us happy. Cool and the happiness it brings are contextual and impermanent, but we cling to it and the feeling and imagine that we are happy because of the value we attach to the feeling of temperature control.

The Buddhist teachings on attachment say that this is our reaction to everything. We hop from a brief moment of what we think is happiness to the next, with a chasm of despair and craving between each pleasurable encounter. Lama Zopa Rinpoche in *How To Practice Dharma* says: 'For most of us, success in life means success in obtaining the four desirable objects, but actually this is only success in achieving suffering, because desire by its very nature disturbs our mental continuum and causes dissatisfaction.'

Heat and cold are states we physically pass through. Yes, they are visceral, but like the thoughts that plague us during meditation, we can simply choose to observe our reactions to sensation impassively, and not become a player in our own mini-drama as we react and try to reach the sensation that we equate with happiness. I know this is hard to hear, and hard to apply. Happiness is etched in stone in our minds as a result of collecting over our lives the ingredients we are taught create the recipe for a perfect life: love (which comes from another); shelter (which is external to us); wealth (which is never enough); respect and admiration from our community (which is terrifyingly transient). Consider the time it takes to actually achieve and maintain these states across a lifetime. No wonder it is such a struggle for us to find time to meditate and look for our own inner happiness.

Craving Praise/Aversion to Criticism

Most of us don't love being criticised. Primarily because we take criticism so personally and have fixed mindsets where we don't see criticism as a pathway to growth and change. Praise, however, is like a nice big sugar hit where our egos get momentary satiation before crashing back to earth. As a highly unevolved human with a taste for praise, I realised how much of my suffering was linked to craving recognition and praise for what I did. The flipside of this was the fear of what would happen if I lost my status as a 'good girl' and was criticised.

I've discussed in the opening chapters my personal experience of how exhausting and futile the hunt for praise is. Growth mindset is a salve to this eternal striving and hiding from mistakes being found out. By knowing that mistakes lead to growth and attainment of competence, receiving criticism is the step before getting better. Sheryl Sandberg, COO of Facebook, says that the ability to listen to feedback is a sign of resilience. 'I'm giving you these comments because I have very high expectations and I know you can reach them,' is how she ends her performance reviews. She isn't crushing her people, she is offering them the truth, and with it the opportunity for change and strength. When receiving criticism becomes your super power, then you will eagerly seek it. If it's delivered clumsily or feels a little personal, you will be able to see the kindness that lies beneath, or at worst understand the value of the message and lay the rest aside.

Craving a Good Reputation/Aversion to Having Your Reputation Trashed

Craving a good reputation and its inverse—craving to be free from having your reputation destroyed—are the final two worldly dharmas to renounce. When I first read the teaching on the Eight Worldly Dharmas and understood the full extent of my attachment to things, I was deeply shocked. It seemed that everything I wanted and aspired to was one of the eight worldly dharmas. Biggest and most disturbing on the eight worldly dharma hit list for me were the pairings around praise and reputation. I had never considered these as an attachment I suffered from.

Nailing these ones is perhaps trickier than nailing those based on finding happiness in tangible objects. When our happiness and identity are so strongly built on inputs that are external to us, our foundations are understandably shaky at best. The façade, constructed over a lifetime of who we are, linked to what others think and how they reflect their favourable perceptions to us, can be decimated in a matter of minutes. We've all seen the big names and reputations fall from grace, and the difficulty those people ever have in regaining their status. If so much time is spent second-guessing others' reactions to us, then doing nothing is a pretty good way of ensuring that our reputations stay intact.

I think reputational considerations are particularly relevant when you are ascertaining what to do with your life and work. Hopefully by now you will have turned your focus to pursuing a path of alignment with your dharma. A lot of the conflict that arises within ourselves at this time when our true nature of self emerges is in wondering what people are going to think of us when we start our unfolding. Remember the quote at the outset about the greatest regrets of the dying being that they hadn't spent more time doing what they felt was a true expression of who they were? I hazard a guess that if you had asked why these people hadn't acted, the answer would have been at its root a fear of reputational damage and judgement from loved ones or strangers about their choices. When we hand over control to external forces, real or imagined, this is what we get. Indian yogi and poet Sri Aurobindo said, 'The spiritual journey is one of continually falling on your face, getting up, brushing yourself off ... and taking another step.'

You must find courage and humour to undertake the good hustle. In the sage words of author and spiritual teacher Ram Dass: 'I have made a public ass of myself, and what I do is the minute I fall on my face I publicly claim it because I realise that it helps other people and it encourages them to have a willingness to risk in their spiritual work.'

Just sit with that, and imagine the freedom of being an ass and owning it, rather than taking the perpetual airbrush to your life.

Many things about undertaking a spiritual path take what is often described as 'courage'. It sits unchallenged in our language that we need to have extreme levels of bravery to follow our dharma or our paths to our true selves. It would be more helpful if we equally commonly used the expression that it takes fear and cowardice to be tethered to the views and thoughts of other people who themselves are drowning in fear and attachment.

How to Stop Being Human

This idea loops us back to where we started with the childhood question of what we want to be when we grow up. It is a question usually posed by adults with authority and status much greater than ours. The answer to the question always has an explicit or implicit value assignment, which teaches us from a very early age about judgement, approval and disapproval being handed out to us by those who have power over us. And not just our future work choices. It is all forms of our personal expression: our bodies; our sexuality; our choice of friends, of pastimes, faith; of just about whatever.

Shame is instilled and internalised early on, and becomes another form of mental suffering that is used to shut down our yearnings for the life we are drawn to live. Think back across your life to the moments you remember letting go of a dream or aspiration because it didn't fit in with the scheme of things laid out for you. It is well worth revisiting early moments in your life where you had clear moments of happiness and contentment, where you believed you were without limitations. I'm not talking about desire here, I'm talking about the clarity we have as children to somehow see our paths and our truths more clearly, without modifying or second-guessing why we can't do things. I'm not suggesting our parents and teachers redirect us because they want us to live a life of suffering away from our true selves. They do it because it was done to them, and because, through early interventions, they want to stop us from suffering, and because they are terribly afraid of reputational damage for us and for them by proxy. This is the cycle of the eight worldly dharmas that has to be broken in order to achieve happiness, and the achievement of this happiness comes from renouncing life.

Renunciation

How do we renounce life while being in the world? If we are following the Buddhist logic that we have been born into these very specific bodies and lives in Western families and countries (or wherever you are engaging with this text), then we are already in the right place at the right time, so what is so wrong? There is nothing wrong *per se*, as lack of awareness and continuation of that cycle is the reality for most folk. But as you've begun the quest for your dharma, for your happiness, and have opened the door to the question of attachment and suffering through your quest for self-awareness and a path to enlightenment, you may as well get some options on the table as to how to throw off the yoke.

In the teachings of the Buddha, renunciation is renouncing the idea of permanence. If everything is impermanent, including us, our lives and our bodies, then there is nothing to be attached to. Everything changes constantly. When we have no attachment to a state being constant, then the expectation is that no matter what happens, it will be different shortly. Pain or pleasure will both come and go, people and their bodies will come and go, thoughts will come and go, and most certainly you will come and go. So the first tiny steps to renunciation are accepting impermanence and being present to the threat of the eight worldly dharmas derailing our self-discovery through clinging and attachment to stuff.

They aren't going away, it is your relationship with them that is changing and detaching. Even if you were in a cave, or a monastery, suffering and attachment is in the mind, and you can take the worldly dharmas with you. Being in the world is the best place to work on renunciation as there are so many constant reminders of how we are attached and selfish. We are heat-seeking missiles for acknowledgement and praise, and it is here we can make inroads into consciously detaching.

Digital Dharma

One of the most treacherous realms to get caught in the eight worldly dharmas is also one that can be of immense benefit to your good hustle—social media, and the digital landscape more broadly. You've no doubt been working diligently on your digital strategy and how you are going to spread your message virally among all those raging evangelists for your product or service. It's likely to be where you will find your customers and your channels for having meaningful communications, especially in the development of your business pre-launch. Like so many things, the Internet and social media isn't good or bad, it simply is. The value we ascribe to it, however, can turn it from a benign tool for marketing, sales and promotion into a weapon, an addiction and a disaster for your brand and your self.

Where previously our engagement in the sales process was one way, social media gave individuals and groups the chance to speak up and engage in the sales funnel as a two-way experience. The lean start-up principals that are so critical to getting your good hustle started simply couldn't exist without a digital market to release a minimum viable product into, and harvest real-time information and feedback from customers as part of the development cycle. Let me be clear, I'm not a digital denier in any way. I do, however, want to highlight some of the significant dharma downsides of digital as you dive into your good hustle, so you are aware of the hidden traps of being always on. And always on show.

There's no delicate way to put this: social media, especially Facebook, Snapchat and Instagram, are the eight worldly dharma atomic power tools. Want to feel bad about what you don't have? Want to develop social anxiety? Want to feel inadequate in every area of your life? Want to feel you are missing out and overwhelmed simultaneously? Want to curate your every move in fear of getting a negative comment and reap praise? Want to crush people's dreams with the absence of a like? Welcome to the worldly dharmas of Facebook, Snapchat, Instagram and Twitter, instruments that could have been developed solely to superglue people to their egos, fuel attachments and invite commentary from the global self-cherishing peanut gallery.

Social media and its resonance with people across the world is a strong demonstration of the chasm of aloneness that connecting with acquaintances and strangers via a screen can momentarily salve. Channels like Facebook, Snapchat and Instagram allow people to be seen. To feel as though they have an audience and an ear for their lives, some recognition and a constant source of potential approval—and criticism. The very nature of social media is to elicit approval or, by the absence of likes or comments, disapproval. In many cases the two-way feedback mechanism also invites unwelcome and unwarranted criticism, leading to bullying and passive aggressive behaviour. This dramatically modifies the user's capacity to be themselves, speak their truth and live in their dharma—and can cause extreme suffering.

What then is the best way to negotiate the necessary tools that the Internet and social media provide to an emerging entrepreneur? It is very common for the clients I work with to have a deep fear of stepping out on social media, especially with a new product or idea. They are gun-shy from having seen the types of word storms unleashed on celebrities and high-profile businesspeople (usually women) and are frightened that this will be their experience. Happily, this is relatively uncommon.

A more likely pitfall of social media is that it keeps you so easily yoked to the attachments and false perceptions of the eight worldly dharmas. We see social media like a window to the world, where everyone is looking at us critically. It is a domestic peepshow, and we get up every day and perform, with all the inherent performance anxiety that brings. Checking our accounts, looking at everyone else being happy and shiny, tallying up the numbers of likes and comments, noticing with hurt who hasn't liked and commented, or gushing with joy when someone we admire notices us. These are all classic descriptions of the eight worldly dharmas in action. They are also not real; just as Facebook, Instagram, Snapchat, Twitter, and even LinkedIn and the countless new and niche networks that will continue to arise, are built on a fictional snapshot of our lives at a moment in time.

If you are making life transformations, seeking out your dharma path and using digital updates to share your journey with the world, it may feel that you are being especially closely scrutinised by others for a spiritual slip-up. There is also the competition to be the best at playing the role of the spiritual soldier via your social media window—the most uplifting memes, the greenest smoothie, the best shots of you doing vrksasana against an exotic backdrop or retreating with the guru de jour. Boy George put it perfectly in his post-recovery comeback album in the lyric 'My god is bigger than your god'. He beautifully captured the striving that goes on in the name of being holier than thou. The performance of spirituality is quite exhausting and requires a lot of props, which of course cost money and scream attachment. The spiritual bullying that goes on by individuals and businesses that want to help you hit the big time in your new good hustle are unconscionable, using language and campaigns that would put the characters of *Mad Men* to shame. So be alert to this, and by all means use social media as a way to open other people's eyes to the dharma, and to hold yourself accountable to your own commitments. But be aware of the fine line into the ego of wanting to be approved and loved by external parties as you do so.

The constant parade of people's lives, loves, acquisitions and feelings on social media can mean you are committing over and over to building the narrative of who you are for the eyes of others, rather than just being, without the need for approval.

Then there is the time consideration of the digital dharma drama. In the blink of an eye that is our lifetimes, we are increasingly living in a sedentary way, looking at ourselves living our lives through social media posts. Trying to keep up with complimenting, commenting and acknowledging everyone else's daily business is time consuming and exhausting. Especially for the hundreds and thousands of friends and followers you might be trying to manage, rather than the intimate and personal social circle that was once all that was required—and that was hard enough. The irony here is that while we are so busy worrying about our flawless photos and how everyone is looking at us, of course they actually aren't. We, and they, are looking at ourselves—we are looking at our own lack and craving for the things we think we need or are missing through the comparison with others' posts, building craving, aversion, attachment and suffering in the process.

What we think of ourselves is vitally important to the success of any endeavour. However, many times those judgements are not based on who we think we are, but instead fall into the category of 'who others think we are'. We all know that someone else's opinion has minimal actual impact on our daily lives, yet we rely on these imaginary external views to fortify our public profile and actions.

Actor Shirley MacLaine has summed up this preoccupation with external views in a theory she refers to as the 20-40-60 rule. According to Shirley, at twenty, your life revolves around an obsession with what others think of you. At forty, you begin to not care what others think of you. And at sixty, you realise that you really weren't being judged by anyone but yourself. More explicitly, that no one was thinking about anything but themselves the whole time. Shirley says that no matter what our age, we all need to be sixty, and as far as social media goes, she's bang on the money.

How many overweight and stiff people do you think will never do yoga because of the endless images put out by the industry of young, slim, bendy yogis in hotpants with a tropical backdrop? Yoga is the perfect remedy for so many physical and emotional illnesses, yet the barriers to starting to take a class are the perceptions about who does, should do and can do yoga.

The way the yoga industry in the West portrays an ancient science for attaining enlightenment and finding union with the divine through living right is an excellent example of the eight worldly dharmas in digital action. We are conditioned to crave being permanently young, flexible and beautiful, and we have an aversion to being stiff and old. We crave a healthy, flexible body, and we have an aversion to the pain of getting flexible through practice or not being good enough. The end result is we don't go to class, or start a practice, and continue to judge ourselves as not worthy of trying. And because we deny ourselves a tool that can change our lives, we suffer. If any of those feelings are the way you feel about starting your good hustle, creating a life that is full of happiness and fulfilment through being of service, then see it as your dharma to ignore them and get on with the show.

Technology, as I said at the outset, is a neutral tool, there to be used to enhance our capabilities. It is up to us as humans to not be the tail wagged by the mobile device, and to clearly establish in our minds (where else would we do it) our relationship to it. As with everything being endorsed in this book, if the mind is managed, the rest falls into place. Digital tools have to be part of your go-to-market strategy. Depending on what your business idea is, a social media and digital presence may be your entire business strategy. Again, we are creating a space as good hustlers living in the world, and the world, including the digital world, is where we are trying to effect our change. We need to be part of the ways of the world and the people we want to connect with.

How do you actually feel when you spend minutes (and, cumulatively, hours) scrolling through other people's cataloguing of the eight worldly dharmas? As an exercise in awakening, hang out on your social media channels and start to classify each post: is it displaying material things or comfort (such as new purchases, gifts, friends, food, booze, holidays, pets and kids) or good reputation and praise (such as new jobs, awards, achievements and recognition by authorities in the sector)? Take the time to recognise how much of the display of social media is the embodiment of the eight worldly dharmas, and how this makes you feel.

When you are auditing the posts think to yourself: do I need to respond? Does it make me want to post up my own picture by way of self-validation? Does it fuel my attachments? In an objective and compassionate view, how many of these posts really matter, or take me closer to self-realisation or my own dharma? I'm not asking you to trawl through and trash all of your friends for their attachments (because as we are all one, they are simply being us, right?). I'm asking you to apply a different lens to an activity that all of us spend a lot of our precious and limited time in. Time to do a little renunciation, and to revisit the eight limbs of yoga in this exercise to remind yourself of stilling down, cleansing the mind, turning in, connecting and finding union. And stay sixty.

The Internet and all of the broader applications of technology that have emerged from it are a boon for connectivity, for information sharing, for showing people that their tribes exist and they are not alone in their thoughts and beliefs. It is an irreversible change to how we do business and communicate, and it can be your best tool in reaching out and finding the people who it is your dharma to connect with through your good hustle. All good. Take the time to readjust your lens on your own attachments (here's a tip, this could take a while) and bring your new vision to your social media interactions. If it is taking up too much time and emotional space in your life, pull back. Post mindfully, stop looking for praise and validation, actively don't use your channels as a way to stay caught in the eight worldly dharmas. Use social media as a space to serve others and genuinely connect with love and compassion.

The social trivia of endless news feeds is the trash that we are filling our brains with. These are the irritating and invasive thoughts that bounce up and down in our minds while we are trying to settle into our meditation. I think sometimes our minds in meditation just look like a rolling social media feed as we play through our catalogue of wants and wishes, fears and hates. I'm not saying throw the baby out with the bathwater. I'm saying that the water needs to be purified through stillness, letting the mud settle to the bottom so the lotus can grow.

If you can use all your restraints of meditation to engage and lovingly observe the flow of attachment on social media without desire, craving, aversion and suffering—great. If not, it might be time to employ some renunciation tactics and reallocate the time. I have a friend who is a psychotherapist and a Buddhist who uses social media as part of his business. He has a strict practice of digital engagement, working on his business in the morning after his meditation practice, scheduling posts, writing blogs and responding to people. In winter, when he sees the sky turn darker earlier and his clients get more introspective and affected by the cooler weather, he initiates a total social media hibernation from his personal social media channels, not looking or responding, except for business reasons. This is his version of digital renunciation and retreat. He is turning inwards from the madness of attachment in the world and removing that distraction and junk from the mind. I think it is a great strategy for everyone, and an important stake in the ground to remind ourselves that our lives and the lives of others have meaning outside of the digital domain. We just have to get out there and remember that the good hustle is a lived experience, both in mind and body.

Social media is an excellent place to observe the eight worldly dharmas in action, and your interaction with them—especially your attachment to reputation and praise. The advent of social media was undoubtedly up there with the Industrial Revolution and mass land and air transport in terms of the transformation it created in how, when and where we do business. It gave us the capacity to connect through lines of shared interest, created communities and began to move information at speeds never before experienced. One of its most critical uses was and is connectivity, the reimagining of society and community along digital lines rather than geographical ones. It literally opened up the world to us, and in doing so, created (somewhat) a democratisation of information and voices.

With all change there is disruption and collateral damage. As Arjuna was all too aware in Gita's battle of Kurukshetra, the battle would kill millions of people and sentient beings, but as Krishna so persuasively argued, it was necessary for the battle to happen, and for Arjuna's dharma to be a part of it.

The Beginning of the End

Writer Elizabeth Gilbert's thesis in her book *Big Magic*, which I cited lovingly earlier, is that creative ideas call you, and if you aren't ready for the call, they will eventually move on and lodge with someone else who is ready to execute. This isn't a good or bad thing, it is simply a thing, and giving the ideas a vehicle to emerge from is part of the human condition. She could well have been talking about dharma, as throughout your life your dharma will have popped its head up in the form of opportunities or windows into another world that you may have chosen to take, or looked wistfully through before turning back to what you were doing.

I like this idea of creativity striking humans, and recognise the transience and impermanence of the visitation. One thing that is a feature of all, and I mean all, start-up business successes I have seen is timing. And not the type of timing where you have all of the dominoes set out in an elaborate, complex pattern, and at the perfect moment you release the marble that tips them into a spectacular cascade. It is a timing that appears completely random, and is the timing of opportunity meeting the market at the same time as you are ready to be the vehicle that makes it all happen. Your readiness to hear the call *and* take the action is the single most important part of success, and it is very un-plannable. Your capacity to act, however, comes from preparation. If you are training for a marathon, you would have run long distances for weeks if not months in the lead-up to the point you actually run the marathon. All of the work you do through the eight limbs of the Yoga Sutras, the mind management, and renouncing of attachment of the eight worldly dharmas, is your training. The self-study and self-sacrifice for the big race of living in your dharma is all work towards the moment when suddenly it is on, when opportunity and market demand appear from nowhere, and you need to lace up your shoes and go. You will know what the call is. You can have some pre-race chat with your trusted guides and mentors, but ultimately, the call to go is yours, and you need to not get waylaid by your own or others' fears of whether it is the right or wrong thing to do. There is no ideal time, but there is a right time. All of your practice and rigour to prepare your mind will kick in like rote at that moment.

You won't hesitate, you'll just say yes and go. As Krishna says to Arjuna in the Gita over and over in different ways: when you know who you are, you will know how to act.

Gandhi practised the mantra of repeating 'Ram' over and over throughout his life, no matter what he was doing, no matter where he was. He had taken on the advice Krishna gave in the Gita to constantly repeat a holy name wholeheartedly, and Lord Ram was the name he chose. In doing so, his mind was turned to the divine and he knew that whatever happened, he was surrendered and ready for a good death. When he was fatally shot in the heart, as he looked his assailant in the eyes and fell to the ground, he uttered the words 'Ram, Ram', such was his training in keeping his mind focused. In the Buddhadharma, it is believed that whatever your mind is set on in your last moments, this is the determinant as to how your next life will be. All the actions of this life are pointed towards a peaceful, happy death and attaining another human rebirth so you can continue to work towards the enlightenment of all through your selfless service.

If you are constantly working to be living in your dharma, and open to how, when and where that might play out, you are creating the single-pointed environment for this to happen. When it does, you will be perfectly ready to say yes and begin. More importantly, the practice of the practice will mean that everything you do is dharma focused, and mindful, and surrendered, and strategically aligned with renouncing attachment to the eight worldly dharmas. So you will already, in theory, be living in service. Love, serve and remember your dharma—a simple mantra that will serve you well as you begin this journey through yourself to yourself.

Following your dharma into a good hustle doesn't mean that life will be without suffering or hardship. Happiness isn't about an absence of challenge, it is about a surplus of acceptance. As Stephen Cope says in his book *The Great Work of Your Life: A Guide for the Journey to Your True Calling*, dharma saves us not by ending, but by redeeming, our suffering. It enables us to bear our suffering, and most importantly, it enables our suffering to bear fruit for the world. For Stephen Cope, meeting the dharma in your life is not about a big, grand gesture of doing, of the fame and fortune that we are groomed through the media to believe is everyone's destiny for at least fifteen minutes. It is about realising that the thing you do, which is *your* thing that is completely aligned with your true self, is often small and composed. Most importantly, it is yours, and the one place where we have the opportunity to discover our true selves.

Epilogue

It's time to have big thoughts,
huge thoughts!
All the conditions are there.
What we need now is the
determination to do it.

LAMA ZOPA RINPOCHE, BUDDHIST TEACHER

I hope this book has inspired you to look deeper into your own existence, your reason for being here. I hope it has awakened in you the recognition that what you are looking for exists, and the idea that you can access it as soon as you try. I'm not sugarcoating: good hustling is hard and is not a fast-food quick fix. There is no fixed destination. But it is a levelling-up of daily joy and meaning. I'm sure you've repeatedly heard it said that happiness comes from within, and been left frustrated and wondering whether your within is broken. The memes and truisms of self-help only give you the large print. They don't often tell you that the work takes a lifetime of days. It's austerity, renunciation and sacrifice, and deep personal investigation. You will gently let go of friends, of jobs, perhaps of partners and family members, of pastimes and activities that used to fire you up momentarily. At the same time you will find new friends quietly fall in line, that old ones who know you so well grow with you; you will see a deepening of existing love, and revelations of support that will fire your resolve like a kiln.

You will find courage you never knew existed, humour, grace and wisdom you had denied you possessed. Use that wisdom to remind yourself that even a moment of peace, a minute of looking your true self in the eye with love, an hour of feeling connected to a vast expanse of sentient beings, makes your life worth it all. Your being belongs to the world, your dharma is calling you to action. Meet it halfway, fall in love with it. And yourself.

The good hustler in me sees and acknowledges the good hustler in you, and together we say 'Namaste'.

Further Reading

Ed Catmull *Creativity Inc.: Overcoming the Unseen Forces that Stand in the Way of True Inspiration*

Stephen Cope *The Great Work of Your Life: A Guide for the Journey to Your True Calling*

Stephen Cope *The Wisdom of Yoga*

Krishna Das *Chants of a Lifetime*

Ram Dass *Be Here Now*

Ram Dass *Paths to God: Living the Bhagavad Gita*

Angela Duckworth *Grit: The Power of Passion and Perseverance*

Professor Carol Dweck *Mindset: The New Psychology of Success*

Eknath Easwaran *The Bhagavad Gita*

Ana Forrest *Fierce Medicine*

Gandhi *An Autobiography: The Story of My Experiences With Truth*

Gandhi *The Bhagavad Gita According to Gandhi*

Elizabeth Gilbert *Big Magic: Creative Living Beyond Fear*

Chris Guillebeau *The $100 Startup*

Tony Hseih *Delivering Happiness*

B.K.S. Iyengar *Light on Life*

B.K.S. Iyengar *Light on the Yoga Sutras of Patanjali*

Vicki Mackenzie *Cave in the Snow*

Mark Manson *The Subtle Art of Not Giving a F*ck*

Abraham H. Maslow 'A Theory of Human Motivation'

Tenzin Palmo *Into the Heart of Life*

Swami Prabhupada, *Bhagavad Gita As It Is*

Eric Reis *The Lean Start-up*

Lama Zopa Rinpoche *How To Practice Dharma*

Lama Zopa Rinpoche *Transforming Problems into Happiness*

Sheryl Sandberg and Adam Grant *Option B: Facing Adversity, Building Resilience, Finding Joy*

Chögyam Trungpa *Cutting Through Spiritual Materialism*

Chögyam Trungpa *Work, Sex, Money: Real Life on the Path of Mindfulness*

Bronnie Ware *The Five Top Regrets of the Dying*

Acknowledgements

No book is an island, especially when you live on one. *The Good Hustle*, like all ideas that make it through execution and into the market, was a collaboration of smarts with heart, and I am extremely grateful to everyone who played a part in its evolution.

The whole team at Murdoch Books are a dream to work with, and taught me so much about the process of being an author along the way. Big props especially to Lou Johnson, Katie Bosher, Madeleine Kane, Vivien Valk, Romina Panetta, Louise Cornege, Jemma Crocker, Henrietta Ashton (who named the puppy), plus all the loving hands from Murdoch and Allen and Unwin globally that touched the manuscript on its way to the bookstore. My deepest Namaste.

Writing is the easy part, the hard part is in the edit. Editor Meaghan Amor is well named, as she is love personified for an author, with a prescient eye, firm but fair touch on the delete button, and a structural knack that is a boon from the gods. Thank you, from the bottom of my grammatically challenged, wordy heart.

The writer's ego is fragile, and while words can be defended, it takes a brave soldier to take the profile shots. To the master of the lens Douglas Frost, thanks, you always make me as pretty as brutalist architecture.

Before it even got to the doors of Murdoch, there was a dedicated group of gals who put the text through its paces, and took the time to smash through the unedited first cut, diligently annotating what they loved and what made them go hmmmm. Reading a big, rambling document is torture, so to Zoe Coyle, Suse Henshaw, Rachel Treasure, Helen Cushing, Tanya Trost, Emily Hassett, Julie Regan and my travelling muse Clare Dunne, what you did validated and refined my vision, and each of you are woven into the pages like beautiful strands of DNA. To the Krishna Village yogis Lila Kirtana, Henrike Schreer and Mal Knights, thank you for keeping me bhakti and bendy in mind and body.

And finally, to Roisin McCann, thank you for tipping the first domino on my path to publication.

FEAR ROBS US OF BEING IN THE PRESENT.
WE ARE LIVING IN OUR MINDS
IN AN UNKNOWN PLACE AND TIME,
FIGHTING BATTLES THAT HAVEN'T STARTED
WITH ADVERSARIES WHO DON'T EXIST.

Dr Polly McGee is an author, entrepreneur educator, digital strategist and yogi.

As co-founder of Start-up Tasmania, she was voted one of the most influential people in Australian start-ups. She has worked with hundreds of start-ups to help them refine their business ideas and connect with their markets.

A prolific speaker and writer on digital strategy and small business, Polly contributes to a range of publications and has created a suite of digital and video content and workshops. She continues to coach heart-centred entrepreneurs, helping them scale their businesses to make a greater impact in the world.

She is strongly committed to the good hustle and believes all of life's problems can be solved with yoga and meditation, and by patting retired greyhounds.

Also by Polly McGee:
Dogs of India

pollymcgee.com
Instagram: @pollymcgee
Twitter: @pollymcgee